The CareWise Guide

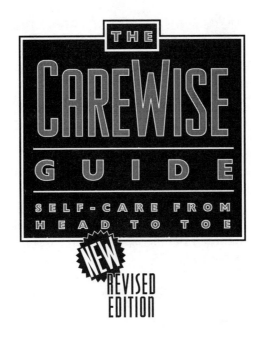

Second Edition

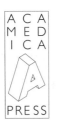

Acamedica Press
A division of EMC^2 (Employee Managed Care Corporation)
Seattle, Washington
1996

Reviewed for medical accuracy by the
College of Physicians and Surgeons of Columbia University
New York, New York

The CareWise Guide: Self-Care From Head To Toe
Second Edition

Published by
Acamedica Press
A division of
EMC² (Employee Managed Care Corporation)
PO Box 34570
Seattle, Washington 98124-1570

Library of Congress Catalog Card Number 96-083132

ISBN 1-886444-01-3

Published 1996
Printed in the United States of America

10 9 8 7 6 5 4 3 2

Medical information in this book was reviewed for accuracy by the College of Physicians and Surgeons of Columbia University and was found to be consistent with generally accepted medical practices at the time of review.

The CareWise Guide is intended to provide general information on common medical topics. It is not a comprehensive medical text and does not include all the potential medical conditions that could be represented by certain symptoms. Therefore, it cannot and should not be relied upon as a substitute for seeing an appropriate health care professional.

Acamedica Press has made every effort to print trademarked product names within this book in initial capital letters to indicate trademark and/or registered trademark designation.

CareWise®

Where to find what you need

A COMPLETE TABLE OF CONTENTS BEGINS ON PAGE XI.

Turn to the first page of each section for specific topics and their page numbers. See the index, pages 391 to 422, for terminology and references as well as specific topics.

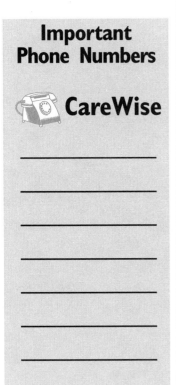

Important Phone Numbers

CareWise

_____

_____

_____

_____

_____

_____

_____

PAGES

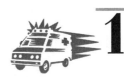

Helping You Make Wise Health Care Decisions

ACKNOWLEDGMENTS

We wish to acknowledge the many medical and communications professionals who contributed to the publication of *The CareWise Guide* including:

Editorial Staff
Randi Holland, RN
Ginny Smith
Sherry Stoll, MSN, RN, CNA
Douglas Weiss
Diane Volk Young

Research and Review Staff
Cynthia Collette, RN; Judy Dundas, RN, BSN; Robin L. Fendick, RN, BSN; Debbie Jepson, RN; Shelby Platt; Margo Sturgis, RN, GNP

Outside Support
Contributing writers
Peg Carver, Jennie Krull Gulian, Robert Miskimon,
Kip Richards, MN, RN

Layout and illustration/Confluence Communications
Production/Darrel Young Design
Cover and page design/Digital Ink Corporation
Illustration/Woodcox Advertising and Communications
Proofreading services/The Write Stuff, Inc.

Medical research provided in part by Reliance Medical Information, Inc., Greenwich, Connecticut.

We appreciate the assistance of Thomas Q. Morris, MD, who coordinated Columbia University's review process.

Special thanks to our many members who are helping us continually improve our quality of services and who are taking the initiative for their own health.

TO HELP YOU WORK IN PARTNERSHIP WITH YOUR DOCTOR

The CareWise Guide is not intended to take the place of your doctor or other health care professionals. It is a resource to help you make the best decisions and get the *most* from the medical services available to you.

Contents

Abdominal/Gastrointestinal

Muscles/Bones/Joints

Women's Health

Preface

Helping you make wise health care decisions

Managing your own health and that of your family is undoubtedly one of your primary concerns. So it should be especially comforting to know that — through CareWise — you have convenient access to health care information and the support you need to make the best possible decisions.

The CareWise Guide is your key resource. It provides you with the best available health care information to help you decide when to apply self-care, when to seek medical care, and how to work effectively with your doctor to get the most appropriate, cost-effective and highest quality health care.

This book is also a tool to help you take charge of your own health and the health of your family. Its focus is on self-care — making healthy lifestyle and preventive decisions, understanding your symptoms and medical concerns, participating with your doctor in shared decision making, and effectively managing your medical conditions.

The information in this book is the result of hundreds of thousands of interactions between CareWise Nurses and individuals just like you. Every week, thousands of CareWise members call our registered nurses for help with medical concerns ranging from sore throats to cancer, from sports injuries to back surgery. No question is too simple or too sensitive.

We have taken this extensive experience, combined it with leading sources of health and medical information, and presented the material in an easy-to-understand format. The medical information has been developed by physicians, nurses and health educators in response to consumers' needs, and reviewed for accuracy by the College of Physicians and Surgeons of Columbia University.

Our goal is to help you become *care-wise*, which means getting in the habit of weighing the benefits, risks and costs when it comes to your specific medical concern. As you do, you will experience better health, greater satisfaction when you seek medical care, and — in the end — the highest quality care.

Health care decisions are personal and important, and they can have a tremendous impact on your overall well-being. *The CareWise Guide* is written to give you the information you need to take charge of your health — from head to toe.

Introduction

Taking charge

Your health is in your hands

In today's rapidly changing world of health care there is one certainty — what you do to maintain or improve your health has a much greater impact on your quality of life than advances in medical science and the treatment of disease.

The most effective ways to reduce disease and disability are those that address your lifestyle and personal health practices. You might be surprised to know that your lifestyle accounts for 53% of what impacts your health, while medical care impacts only 10%*. In fact, nine out of 10 of the leading causes of death are preventable, and personal responsibility truly is the key to good health.

Why is it, then, that we too often leave the state of our health in the hands of fate, doctors or genetics and remain passive participants? Why are we content to avoid illness rather than concentrating on becoming healthier? Simply put, we have the *desire* to be healthy, but lack the skills and information we need to *take charge*.

The goal of *The CareWise Guide: Self-Care From Head To Toe* is to help you develop the confidence to manage your medical concerns — from becoming a knowledgeable consumer of services to staying as healthy as possible.

A self-care approach

There is a common misconception that healthy living is hard work. In truth, an effective self-care approach is much easier and more rewarding than falling into poor health and having to work your way back to good health.

A successful self-care strategy has three key ingredients: prevention, participation and education.

PREVENTION

Making healthy lifestyle and preventive decisions can have an enormous impact on reducing your risk of disease. The best place to start is with the behaviors that can make the biggest difference.

The Wellness for Life Workbook

Taking steps to exercise regularly, eat a healthy diet, quit smoking, reduce your alcohol consumption and use of drugs, and control your weight are essential to successful prevention. In addition to your lifestyle choices, immunizations and screening tests can help you prevent health risks, and identify and manage the onset of disease (see *Prevention*, p. 371, to learn more about prevention and recommended immunizations and screenings).

Of course, no amount of prevention can eliminate all disease, which is why your participation in the medical decision-making process is so important.

PARTICIPATION

Unfortunately, our use of medical services is based on the hope that modern medicine will provide a treatment and cure for all our bad habits. The result is that we often overuse medical services for situations we can better handle at home (according to current findings, approximately 80% of all medical concerns can be effectively treated at home). Also, our expectations for medical care often go unmet because we don't fully understand the importance of our own active participation in the decision-making process.

Making participation a part of your self-care strategy means taking charge of *how* you use medical services. This includes understanding your symptoms, making informed decisions about when to seek care, finding the right type of care, and working with your doctor to manage your health.

When you enter your doctor's office with a medical concern, you present a mystery. The more clues you can provide, the quicker your doctor can identify the culprit. Your doctor may be the medical expert, but nobody knows your body like you do. Don't hesitate to offer information and ask questions (see *Becoming Partners With Your Doctor*, p. 385, for more tips on how to work with your doctor).

EDUCATION

When it comes to the health of you and your family, ignorance is not bliss. Learning what your self-care options are — when it is safe to treat health problems at home — and when to see a doctor saves everyone time and money. Being educated means sidestepping unnecessary treatment and testing, avoiding extra medical charges, and requesting generic drugs when they are less expensive but just as effective as name brands.

Most importantly, working to improve your health and decrease your need for medical services is critical to solving our national concern over the cost of health care. You and your family can improve the quality of care you receive by combining it with a self-care approach — becoming part of the solution rather than part of the problem.

What is CareWise?

The CareWise Guide is part of a unique benefit called CareWise. CareWise is a comprehensive health care information service specifically designed to give you and your family the information, support and guidance you need to make wise health care decisions. In our experience with over a million CareWise members, we know that when you are sick or worried you may want more than a written resource.

CareWise registered nurses are available by phone, 24 hours a day, seven days a week, to help you understand your medical concerns, evaluate self-care options and even prepare questions for your doctor. They can research your options, send you information, coach you on how to make your doctor appointments more productive, and help you understand how "managed care" affects your decisions.

Individuals who use CareWise take more responsibility for their own health and use of medical services. They report that they are more knowledgeable about their decisions and more comfortable working in partnership with their doctor. As a result of CareWise and their self-care approach, CareWise members experience a noticeable improvement in the quality of care they receive and a decrease in the time and money they spend on health care.

Answers to some commonly asked questions

Q. *How do I decide whether my problem is important enough to call CareWise?*

A. Any health problem that is troubling you — no matter how silly or insignificant you may think it seems — is worth a call to CareWise.

Q. *What kinds of things do people call about?*

A. Just about any health problem you can think of. For example: "I just found out my cholesterol level is sky-high. How can I get it under control?" "My kids have chicken pox." "I want to stop smoking." "When I left my doctor's office I had more questions than when I went in."

Q. *Will you tell my employer or insurance carrier that I've called CareWise?*

A. All calls are confidential unless you have signed a release form with your employer or insurance carrier granting them access to your medical information. While we will ask for your name and the member identification number of the eligible CareWise member, we will only use that information to determine your eligibility and establish a medical chart for you.

6 tips for putting CareWise to good use

1. Keep *The CareWise Guide* in a spot where everyone in your family can find it quickly and often.

2. Browse the guide *before* you or a family member is sick or injured. Find out the kind of information it contains and where to find what you need.

3. Make sure your family knows how to use *The CareWise Guide* and how to call CareWise if they have additional questions or concerns.

4. Have the Social Security number of the eligible CareWise member ready when you call CareWise.

5. **Don't call CareWise in an emergency situation.** Call 911 or your local emergency services number.

6. Remember that no question or problem is too insignificant for CareWise. Just call!

Using The CareWise Guide

Finding what you need

Let's say it's 1 a.m. and your four-year-old has a fever. Or it's Sunday afternoon and you've pulled a muscle playing volleyball. You're wondering whether to call your doctor or just wait. The problem is, you need help — now!

Open up *The CareWise Guide: Self-Care From Head To Toe*, a book that's designed to serve as your around-the-clock health care guide.

The CareWise Guide covers close to 200 topics, ranging from measles to menopause, from appendicitis to varicose veins. We suggest you take a few moments, now, to browse through the book and familiarize yourself with its format and contents. We think you'll discover that it's filled with helpful information about all kinds of common, day-to-day health concerns — like what to do if your child has an ear infection or a fever, or if you have a funny-looking mole, or suddenly hurt your back or sprain your ankle.

Most topics include general information about the medical problem, as well as tips for:

• Prevention

• Treating the problem at home

• When to seek professional medical care

Where to find what you need

- **Emergencies and injuries** are covered at the beginning of the book — where they are readily accessible. **In case of an emergency, call 911 or your local emergency services number. CareWise is not designed to be an emergency or urgent care service.**

- **Chief concerns** come next, and are organized in a head-to-toe fashion — beginning with neurological problems and working all the way through the body, right down to foot and toe pain. (In addition to the table of contents, see the reference chart on page v to quickly find various topics.) The detailed index in the back of the book is designed to help you look up specific words and references and direct you to related topics.

  Other important sections include Infant/Child Health, Medications, Prevention and Working With Your Doctor.

- *Know What To Do* **sections,** which accompany most topics, are designed to help you decide when self-care is appropriate, when to call a doctor, and when to apply emergency first aid and seek emergency aid. Read on for details on how to use the *Know What To Do* sections.

Using the *Know What To Do* sections

- First, read all the general information about the topic. It will help you better understand *Know What To Do*.

- Next, work your way through *Know What To Do*. Don't skip from point to point; each point is based on the assumption that you have answered yes or no to the previous one. Follow the arrows that apply to each of your answers.

- Take action based on the yes arrow that most appropriately applies to your health concern. Or, if *Know What To Do* refers you to another topic in the book, you can turn to that page for additional information. For example, *Know What To Do* for nausea and vomiting tells you to "see *Dehydration*, p. 262" for details on that particular side effect of nausea and vomiting.

What does each action step mean?

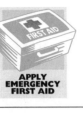

APPLY EMERGENCY FIRST AID

Begin emergency first aid **immediately**.

SEEK EMERGENCY CARE

Get professional medical help **immediately**.

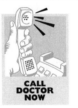

CALL DOCTOR NOW

Call your doctor's office **now** and alert the doctor — or a nurse — to the problem. Ask them what you should do next. This is a situation that needs prompt, professional attention, but is not necessarily an emergency.

CALL DOCTOR

Phone your doctor's office today and talk to the doctor or a nurse about the problem. Make an appointment if it's decided that it's necessary.

APPLY SELF-CARE

Follow the directions for self-care (listed in the *What You Can Do* section) carefully. If you become worried about your condition, call your doctor or CareWise.

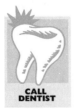

CALL DENTIST

Phone your dentist's office today and talk to the dentist about the problem.

Need more details?

After reading the section(s) covering your medical concern, you may have questions and want additional information. A CareWise Nurse is just a phone call away and is ready to help you understand your situation, provide additional medical information, evaluate options for care or help you develop questions for your doctor.

Just call!

The CareWise Guide is not intended to take the place of your doctor or other health care professionals. Instead, it is a resource to help you make the best decisions and get the *most* from the medical services available to you.

CareWise success stories

You're taking charge — with remarkable results!

If you are like most of us, you have lived your life believing that the realm of health care is well beyond your understanding and control, and that your role as a patient is to passively follow your doctor's orders — no questions asked.

Well, CareWise members are consistently proving that these old beliefs are not necessarily true. In fact, many of you are experiencing remarkable results as you begin to take more control of your own health. Here are just three examples.

"The CareWise Guide told us exactly what to do!"

"It was about three in the morning and suddenly she was jerking, her jaw was clenched and her eyes were locked in a stare!" says Bonnie. Her 18-month-old daughter, Kate, was having a febrile seizure. In spite of their terror, she and her husband, Mark, were prepared and knew what to do.

"Kate had an ear infection and was running a fever of 103° F," says Bonnie. "I'd heard somewhere that babies with fevers sometimes have convulsions, so at least I knew what was happening when it started." What's more, Bonnie and Mark had spent some time browsing *The CareWise Guide.*

Bonnie raced for the self-care guide and flipped to the section on self-care for convulsions, while Mark stayed with the baby. "It said to time the length of the convulsion, so I looked at my watch and wrote down the time," says Bonnie. "The book also said that febrile seizures in young children aren't usually a serious problem and that helped us stay a little calmer."

Step by step, Bonnie and Mark followed the guide's instructions. "We rolled Kate on her side to drain out saliva so she wouldn't choke, and didn't put anything between her teeth. We couldn't have anyway because her jaw was locked so tight!" says Bonnie.

When the seizure ended about three minutes later, they put a cool washcloth on Kate's forehead and checked the guide to decide whether to call their pediatrician.

"The book said to call after the seizure ended," says Bonnie. They did, and were told to get Kate's fever down and then bring her in. "We put her in a bath, gave her some Tylenol, and were in the emergency room by about 5 a.m.," says Bonnie.

Happily, the doctor confirmed that Bonnie and Mark had done everything right and that Kate was going to be fine. "Now that she's had one seizure she's more likely to have them again, but at least we know what they are and we know what to do," says Bonnie. "If it wasn't for *The CareWise Guide,* we wouldn't have had a clue. We probably would have thought Kate was dying!"

"My doctor said I needed surgery and I said no way!"

Judy's car accident is still vivid in her mind. "I saw the other car coming and there wasn't anything I could do but just sit, gripping the steering wheel," she says.

After the crash, the pain in her left hand and arm "sometimes would wake me up at night, shooting from my wrist up to my shoulder," says Judy. "It was like someone sticking pins into me."

But pain was just the beginning of her problems. "I started having trouble writing and picking up things," remembers Judy, whose job involves working at a computer — all day, every day. "My hand and arm hurt even more when I gripped something. Then one day I tried to lift a gallon of milk and dropped it. That's when I knew something was really wrong."

For six months Judy searched for help, going from one doctor to the next, with physical therapy and diagnostic tests in between. Finally, her primary care physician diagnosed her with a nerve problem and sent her to a neurologist. He said she needed surgery and would have to be off work for six weeks.

"I can't afford to miss that much work, and there's no way I want an operation!" says Judy. It was the threat of surgery that prompted her to pick up *The CareWise Guide* and call a CareWise Nurse.

"The nurse explained everything to me, and together we read through the section on carpal tunnel syndrome in *The CareWise Guide*," says Judy. "She helped me come up with questions to ask my doctor — including whether there were other ways to treat the problem besides surgery." For example, she suggested that Judy ask about anti-inflammatory medication and wearing a splint, "which I never would have known about."

Judy went back to her doctors, who agreed to try medication before going ahead with surgery. "Sure enough, the medicine worked wonders and the pain is much better," says Judy. "It hurts every now and then, but — by using medication when the pain flares up, and sleeping in a splint — I'm dealing with it."

Judy says there's still a chance she might consider surgery if the pain gets bad again. "But I'm really glad I didn't rush into anything, and I don't know what I would have done without CareWise. It's such a relief to have someone to talk to about these things."

"I've lost 50 pounds and feel 200% better!"

Tom had a rude awakening the day he heard that his brother was going in for triple-bypass surgery.

"He isn't overweight, he doesn't smoke and he exercises regularly, so I never thought he was a likely candidate for heart disease," says 47-year-old Tom. "On the other hand, heart disease runs in our family and my dad died of a heart attack when he was about 61."

At that point, Tom says he was about 65 pounds overweight, hadn't exercised in years and was a heavy smoker. "I realized that if I wanted to see my 9-year-old daughter grow up, I'd better make some changes — fast!"

Tom went to his doctor for a complete physical and was told that everything checked out fine. "But I was still worried and knew I surely had plenty of room for improvement," he says.

That's when he called CareWise. "The CareWise Nurse answered all my questions about what my cholesterol numbers meant, what risk factors for heart disease are, and sent me information about ways to control cholesterol," he says.

Armed with facts and encouragement from CareWise, Tom began making gradual changes in his lifestyle. For starters, he chose a low-fat, low-cholesterol diet. Then he began exercising.

"I was too out of shape and smoked too much to start out fast, so I began walking around the school track a couple times a day, at a normal pace. I worked my way up to three and then four laps, and then I started increasing my pace." Within five months, he was speed-walking five to seven miles a day.

Tom also started exercising at home, on a minitrampoline. "When I started I could only do two or three minutes at a time, but I gradually worked my way up to 30 minutes a day."

Today, just eight months after launching his self-improvement program, Tom has lost 50 pounds. "I feel 200% better — like a whole new person — and I have energy to spare," he says. "Sure, I still have a ways to go, but I can definitely see light at the end of the tunnel." Tom wants to lose another 10 or 15 pounds and quit smoking. "I can hardly wait to see how much better I feel after I give up cigarettes!" he says.

Tom is quick to offer encouragement to others who want to make lifestyle changes. "Just remember that you're never too old and it's never too late. If I can do it, anyone can!"

Case studies are based on real CareWise experiences. Names and other details have been changed to maintain confidentiality.

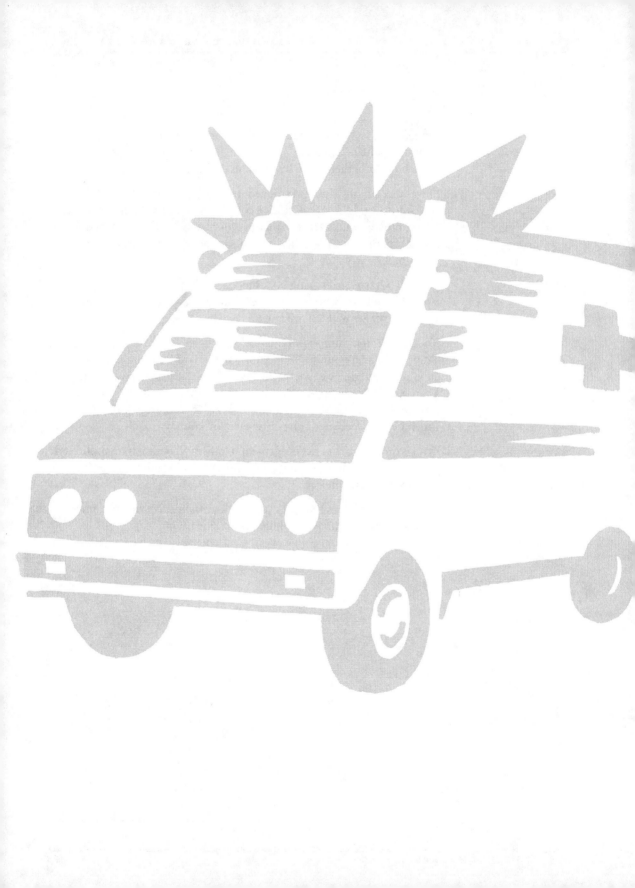

Emergencies 1

READER'S NOTE:

For every medical concern covered in *The CareWise Guide*, you'll find information that will help you determine whether you have an emergency. Look for this symbol.

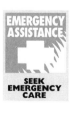

EMERGENCY ASSISTANCE

SEEK EMERGENCY CARE

Emergencies

No time for panic

The time to prepare for a medical emergency is now — not at the scene of a car accident or on the doorstep of someone who is having a heart attack.

An emergency by definition is an unexpected occurrence that demands immediate action. Staying calm — rather than panicking — is the key, and knowing what to do ahead of time is your best defense against panic.

BE PREPARED

- Write down the phone numbers of the nearest emergency facility, Poison Control Center and rescue squad in the front of this book and your telephone book.

- Know the best way to reach the emergency room by car, in case you need to drive yourself or someone else there.

- Take first-aid and CPR courses. Make both of them family affairs.

- Wear a medical-alert bracelet or necklace or carry emergency medical information in your wallet, especially if you have a condition such as diabetes, epilepsy or serious allergic reactions. This information could save your life if you are unable to speak.

IDENTIFYING AN EMERGENCY

It is sometimes difficult to determine whether a situation is an emergency. But if you think symptoms seem critical or life-threatening, then the victim probably should be taken to an emergency room.

These symptoms usually indicate an emergency situation:

- A serious wound (see *Wounds*, p. 46) or broken bone (see *Broken Bones*, p. 75)

- No pulse or breathing (see *CPR*, p. 20)

- Unconsciousness (see *Unconsciousness*, p. 40)

- Active bleeding (see *Control Severe Bleeding*, p. 47)

- Signs of a heart attack (see *Chest Pain*, p. 218)
- Disorientation in someone who has previously been alert
  (see *Shock*, p. 42)

If possible, call ahead to the emergency room to allow emergency personnel to prepare for your arrival. Explain the nature of the victim's problem and provide the name and phone number of the victim's doctor.

WHEN TO CALL AN AMBULANCE

Although it is always important to err on the side of safety, make sure you have a true emergency before calling an ambulance or aid car. It is expensive and the medical assistance may be needed more somewhere else.

Generally, an aid car with paramedics is needed if the victim has:

- Symptoms of a heart attack (severe chest pain, shortness of breath, sweating)
- Severe breathing problems
- Possible spinal, neck or head injury (**do not attempt to move the victim yourself**)
- Severe bleeding

Cardiopulmonary resuscitation (CPR)

Prepare by taking a course

CPR is an emergency first-aid technique for treating a person who is not breathing and has no heartbeat.

This is a skill that is most often used by friends and family members on each other. That's why it's a good idea to encourage each member of your household to learn the techniques.

When it's needed, the person who has the most experience and training in CPR should be the one to perform the procedure at the scene of an emergency.

THINK ABC — AIRWAY, BREATHING AND CIRCULATION

In basic life support, remember ABC:

- **A**irway - Establish an open airway
- **B**reathing - Reestablish breathing
- **C**irculation - Begin external compressions if the heart has stopped

Step one — Check for consciousness/Call for help:

- Find out if the person is conscious. Shout, "Are you OK?"
- Move the victim only if necessary. Gently roll them over onto their back, keeping the head, neck and shoulders together as a unit. If you suspect a spinal injury, be careful not to move the victim's neck.
- If the victim doesn't respond, call 911 or your local emergency services number, then begin CPR, if necessary.
- For children and infants, do one minute of CPR, if indicated, before calling 911 or your local emergency services number.

Cardiopulmonary resuscitation (CPR) is a complex first-aid procedure. Although we describe all the steps for CPR, this section is not intended to replace a course that allows you to have actual hands-on experience with the procedures. To learn CPR, contact the American Red Cross, American Heart Association or other civic groups in your community for classes.

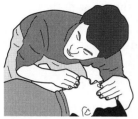

Figure 1

Step two — Check for breathing/Open airway

If no air is passing through the victim's lips (put your cheek next to their mouth to check), and the victim's chest and abdomen are not moving, they are not breathing and you will need to open the airway.

- If there is vomit or liquid in the mouth, clean it out with your fingers (cover fingers with a clean cloth if you have one).

- Push down and back on the forehead and lift up the chin by placing your fingers under the jaw bone.

- With an infant, be careful not to extend the head back too far since that can shut off the airway.

- Check the mouth, chest and abdomen again for movement. Sometimes opening the airway is enough to get the victim to start breathing again.

- If the person does not begin breathing immediately, begin rescue breathing (step three).

Step three — Begin rescue breathing

- Pinch the victim's nostrils shut with the same hand that you have on the victim's forehead (see Figure 1).

- Place your mouth over the victim's mouth, making a tight seal.

- Place your mouth over both the mouth and nose if the victim is an infant. Be careful not to blow too hard into the infant since excess air can go into the stomach and cause vomiting or compression of the lungs. Either one will make delivering air more difficult.

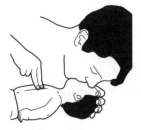

Figure 2

- Slowly blow in air until the victim's chest rises. Remove your mouth between breaths and allow time for the victim to exhale passively before the next breath.

Step four — Check for pulse

- Locate the main (*carotid*) artery in the neck by placing the tips of your index and middle finger on the Adam's apple and sliding them toward your own body into the groove between the *trachea* (windpipe) and the muscles at the side of the neck.

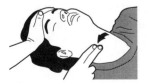

Figure 3

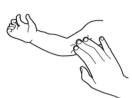

Figure 4

- With an infant, check for the *brachial pulse* on the inside of the upper arm.
- Hold your fingers in place for five to 10 seconds.

IF THERE IS A PULSE

Continue rescue breathing. **Do not do chest compressions on a victim who has a pulse**. CPR performed on a person whose heart is beating can cause serious injury. Instead:

- Blow air into the lungs 12 times per minute (once every five seconds) for an adult and 15 times per minute for a small child (once every four seconds). Breathe 20 times per minute (once every three seconds) for an infant.
- Check the pulse once per minute to make sure the heart is still beating. Continue breathing as long as necessary. A victim who seems to have recovered needs to be seen by a doctor, since shock is a common occurrence after breathing has stopped (see *Shock*, p. 42).

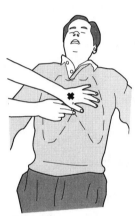

Figure 5

IF THERE IS NO PULSE

Step five: Begin chest compressions

- Find the lower rib cage and move your fingers up the rib cage to the notch where the ribs meet the lower breastbone in the center of the lower part of the chest (see Figure 5).
- Place the heel of one hand down on the breastbone and your other hand on top of the one that is in position. In children 1 to 8 years old, use the heel of one hand rather than both hands.
- Do not compress the chest with your fingers. This can damage the ribs.
- Lock your elbows into position with your arms straight. Place your shoulders directly over your hands so the thrust of each compression goes straight down on the chest.

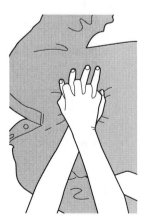

Figure 6

- Push down with a steady, firm thrust, compressing the chest one to two inches for an adult.

- Lift your weight from the victim and repeat. Do not lift your hands from the victim's chest between thrusts.

- Do 15 chest compressions in about 10 seconds.

- After 15 compressions, quickly tilt the head and lift the chin of the victim (as previously instructed), pinch the nose and breathe two slow breaths to fill the lungs. The chest must deflate after each breath.

- Continue this cycle (15 compressions and two breaths) at the rate of 80 - 100 compressions per minute. Check the victim's pulse after one minute. **Continue the compressions and breathing until help arrives if there is still no pulse.**

- For children 1 to 8 years old, compress the chest one to one-half inches and give five chest compressions to one breath.

Extra care must be taken when performing CPR on an infant:

- If chest compression is necessary, position your index and middle fingers on the baby's breastbone.

- Gently compress the chest no more than one inch. Count out loud as you pump in a rapid rhythm — roughly one and a half times a second or about 100 times a minute.

- Gently give one breath (with your mouth covering the baby's mouth and nose) after every fifth compression.

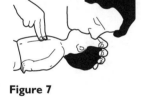

Figure 7

Choking

Quick, simple action can save a life

Thousands of Americans choke to death needlessly every year. People of any age can choke on pieces of food, vomit and small objects.

Prevention

FOR YOURSELF

- Take small bites and chew food thoroughly. Cut meat into small pieces.

- Don't eat too fast, or eat and talk or laugh at the same time.

- Don't drink too much alcohol before eating.

- If you smoke, wait until after you've finished eating to light up.

IF YOU'RE A PARENT OF A SMALL CHILD

- Keep small objects that children might choke on out of reach.

- Do not let children run or jump with food or any other object in their mouth.

- Inspect all toys for small, removable parts that can cause choking. (Follow label guidelines that indicate "appropriate ages.")

What you can do

IF SOMEONE IS CHOKING

You may have only four to eight minutes to save a choking person's life, so you should know how to administer the Heimlich Maneuver (see following pages) and CPR (see *CPR*, p. 20).

A conscious child or adult who is choking will breathe in an exaggerated way. They will be unable to talk or cough, and will probably nod in the affirmative to the question, "Are you choking?" They may grasp their throat. People who can cough or speak are still getting some air into their lungs, and should be encouraged to cough vigorously. The Heimlich Maneuver should not be administered in these cases.

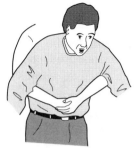

Figure 8

CHOKING RESCUE (HEIMLICH MANEUVER) FOR A CONSCIOUS PERSON

- Establish whether the person can speak or cough by asking, "Are you choking?"
- Stand behind the person.
- Wrap your arms around their waist.
- Grasp one of your fists with the other hand and place the thumb-side of the fist just above the navel but below the rib cage.
- Thrust your fist upward in five quick, sharp jabs.
- Repeat until the object is dislodged or the person becomes unconscious.

CHOKING RESCUE FOR AN UNCONSCIOUS PERSON

- Call 911 or your local emergency services number.
- Check for object in the mouth by sweeping deeply with a hooked finger to remove the object. Use tongue-jaw lift (see Figure 9) and sweep finger to remove object.
- Open airway (push down and back on the forehead and lift up the chin by placing your fingers on the jaw bone). Attempt rescue breathing by pinching the nostrils shut, placing your mouth over the victim's mouth, and giving two breaths. If needed, open the airway and try again.
- If object is still obstructing airway, kneel down and straddle either the person's hips or legs.
- Place the heel of one of your hands against the person's abdomen just above the navel but well below the rib cage, then place your second hand on top of the first.
- Press into the person's abdomen with quick upward thrusts. Do this five times.
- Repeat sequence of finger sweep, rescue breathing attempt and abdominal thrusts until successful or until help arrives.

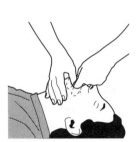

Figure 9

OBSTRUCTED AIRWAY IN CHILDREN 1 TO 8 YEARS OLD

Use same procedure already covered with two important exceptions:
- Look into the airway and use your finger to sweep the object out

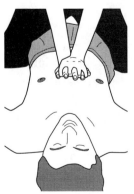

Figure 10

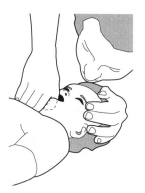

Figure 11

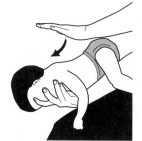

Figure 12

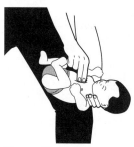

Figure 13

ONLY if you can see it. **DO NOT** perform a blind finger sweep. Instead, perform a tongue-jaw lift (see Figure 11).

- If obstruction is not relieved after one minute, call your local emergency services number. Of course, if someone else is available, have that person call for help immediately. Continue sequence until successful or until help arrives.

OBSTRUCTED AIRWAY IN INFANT OR CHILD LESS THAN 1 YEAR OF AGE

The following steps are appropriate if there is complete airway obstruction due to a witnessed or strongly suspected obstruction by an object. **DO NOT PERFORM these maneuvers to clear an airway that is obstructed due to swelling caused by infection. SEEK EMERGENCY CARE IMMEDIATELY.**

Infant or child is conscious

- Hold infant or child face down along your forearm, supporting the head and neck with one hand.

- Give five back blows forcefully between the shoulder blades with the heel of your hand.

- Turn the infant or child face up. Keeping the head supported and lower than the rest of the body, position your index and middle fingers on the baby's breastbone and give five thrusts with two fingers.

- Do chest thrusts slower than you would for CPR (see *CPR*, p. 20).

- Repeat until the object is dislodged or infant/child is unconscious.

Infant or child is unconscious

- Place the infant or child on a firm surface.

- Open the airway (push down and back on the forehead and lift up the chin by placing your fingers under the jaw bone). With an infant, be careful not to extend the head back too far since that can shut off the airway.

- If victim is not breathing, try to give rescue breaths by covering their mouth and nose with your mouth.

- If unable to give breaths, reposition the head and try again.

- Turn child face down and deliver five back blows (see Figure 12).

- Deliver five chest thrusts.
- Do tongue-jaw lift (see Figure 11). Remove object **ONLY** if you can see it.
- Try again to do rescue breathing.
- Repeat back blows, chest thrusts, tongue-jaw lift and rescue breathing attempts until successful.
- After one minute of emergency first aid, call 911 or your local emergency services number. Of course, if someone else is available, have that person call for help immediately. Continue process until successful or until help arrives.

IF YOU ARE CHOKING AND CAN'T GET HELP

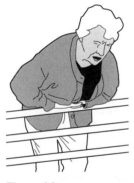

- Try not to panic.
- Cough vigorously.
- If unsuccessful, stand behind a chair or beside or over some other object that puts pressure on your abdomen just above your navel (but below your rib cage).
- Thrust yourself upon the object in strong, sharp bursts.
- Repeat until item is dislodged.

Figure 14

FOR A PREGNANT OR OBESE PERSON

- Stand behind the person and place your arms under their armpits.
- Place fist on the middle of breastbone in the chest, but not over the ribs.
- Place other hand on top of it.
- Give five quick, forceful movements. Do not squeeze with arms, but use your fist.

Final notes

Call your local hospital or Red Cross chapter for more information and instruction on these procedures. **Those who have just had the choking rescue performed on them should see a doctor. The maneuver can cause trauma to the chest or abdomen, and the object may have damaged the throat.**

1

Poisoning

Get help NOW!

**What you
can do**

Call your local Poison Control Center (often listed on the inside front cover of your phone book), hospital or emergency services number **the minute you suspect a poisoning**. Be ready to give the person who answers as much information as possible:

- What substance was taken
- How much
- When
- Victim's age and health status
- Whether victim has vomited
- How far away you are from emergency help

Also immediately: Give the person a glass of milk or water to slow the rate of poison absorption (**DO NOT give them anything to drink if they are unconscious, lethargic or convulsing**).

IF THE PERSON BECOMES UNCONSCIOUS OR STOPS BREATHING

- see *Unconsciousness*, p. 40, or *CPR*, p. 20

IF THE VICTIM IS HAVING CONVULSIONS

- Remove any objects that could cause injury to the person.
- Do not put anything in the person's mouth.

IF YOU ARE INSTRUCTED TO INDUCE VOMITING

- Touch the back of the victim's throat with a finger. If that doesn't cause vomiting ...
- Administer syrup of ipecac, if available, followed by as much liquid as possible. Vomiting will probably begin 15 to 20 minutes later.
- If you do not have syrup of ipecac, use a glass of water with three

teaspoons of salt or one teaspoon of dried mustard.

- Once vomiting begins, make sure the person's head is below chest level to prevent vomit from entering the lungs.

- If vomiting has not begun in 25 minutes, repeat these steps.

If you go to the hospital, take the remains of the suspected poison with you, along with any substance that has been vomited.

NEVER INDUCE VOMITING IF THE PERSON:

- Is unconscious, semiconscious or having a convulsion

- Has a burning sensation in their mouth or throat

- May have swallowed a corrosive agent (dishwasher detergent, bleach, drain opener, oven cleaner, floor wax, grease removers, kerosene, gasoline, clear furniture polish). These substances should be neutralized with milk, water or milk of magnesia.

Prevention

Children ages 1 to 4 years account for 80% of all poisonings. To protect them:

- Never leave children unattended with potentially harmful substances. These include medications, antifreezes, household cleaners, insecticides, organic solvents and fuels.

- Childproof all cupboards with plastic latch locks.

- Keep items in their original containers. This will help your child associate containers and their contents with substances that are off-limits.

- Apply "Mr. Yuk" stickers to containers of poisonous substances, and make sure your child understands their meaning.

- Check walls for peeling paint that a child could rip off and suck. Lead paint is especially dangerous.

- Keep syrup of ipecac available to induce vomiting if needed.

- Teach children where to find and how to use emergency numbers, as well as how to get help in general.

- Post the Poison Control Center telephone number *before* you need to use it.

see *Food Poisoning*, p. 244

Burns

Know how to prevent and treat them

The skin is the body's largest organ, protecting us against infection and helping to regulate the balance of water and temperature. Burns — whether caused by fire, hot objects or fluids, electricity, chemicals, radiation or other sources — threaten these vital functions. For the very young or old, or those with other medical conditions, burns can be even more serious.

Burns are classified based on their depth of penetration of the skin.

- **First-degree** burns involve only the tough, outer layer of skin. The skin turns bright red and becomes sensitive and painful. It may be dry, but it does not blister.

- **Second-degree** burns are deeper than first-degree burns and are very painful, red and mottled. The burned area may blister and/or be swollen and puffy.

- **Third-degree** burns are still deeper and can involve muscle, internal organs and bone. The skin will look charred and dry and may break open. Underlying muscle or tendons may be visible. Pain may be severe. If nerves have been damaged, however, there may be no pain except around edges of the burn.

What you can do

IF SOMEONE IS ON FIRE

- Try not to panic.

- Help the victim drop down and roll in a blanket, rug, coat or some type of covering to smother the flames. Do not let the victim run — this will cause the fire to burn more.

- Completely extinguish the fire and stop skin and clothes from smoldering by soaking with water. Do not remove burned clothing.

- Cover the burn with a cool, damp, sterile bandage or a clean, non-fibrous cloth such as a sheet.

- **Seek emergency care.**

What you can do

FOR SEVERE BURNS OF ANY KIND

Make sure:

- Victim is breathing. If not, **call for emergency help and start CPR immediately** *(see CPR, p. 20)*.

- Bleeding is controlled (see *Control Severe Bleeding*, p. 47).

- There are no signs of shock: altered consciousness, faintness, paleness, rapid and shallow breathing, rapid and weak pulse, cool and clammy skin (see *Shock*, p. 42).

- There are no signs of charring in the mouth or of nasal hairs. Check for sooty residue on the face, shortness of breath, a cough or hoarseness. If present, these signs indicate an emergency; the respiratory tract may be damaged. **Seek emergency care.**

FOR OTHER BURNS

Electrical burns

- Turn off power before touching someone who is in contact with an electrical wire or appliance. Assume a downed power line is live.

- Try not to move the victim.

- If a power line has fallen across a car, passengers remain safest if they stay inside. If they have to leave because of fire or some other reason, they should jump clear of the car.

An electrical burn can appear minor even when it has caused major injuries. There will be wounds at the places of entry and exit of the electrical current which should be evaluated by a doctor.

(See following information on first-, second- and third-degree burns.)

Chemical burns

- Flush the skin with large amounts of cool, running water for 20 minutes or until the burning pain has stopped. If the chemical is a dry solid, brush it off first.

- If an eye has been burned, flush it immediately with lukewarm water. Angle the head so the contaminant does not flow into the other eye. After flushing, close the eye and cover with a loose, moist dressing and **seek emergency care.**

What you can do

- Remove any contaminated clothing, jewelry and other items.
- Cover the area with a cool, damp, sterile dressing or clean cloth and **call your doctor.**

(See following information on first-, second- and third-degree burns.)

First-degree burns

- Run cool water over the area or soak it in a cool-water bath for two to five minutes. If this is not possible, apply cold compresses. (If the burn has occurred in a cold environment, **do not** apply water.)
- Cover the area with a cool, moist, clean bandage or clean cloth.
- Pain relievers — such as aspirin, ibuprofen and acetaminophen (Tylenol) — may help reduce pain and swelling. **NEVER give aspirin to children/teenagers. It can cause Reye's syndrome, a rare but often fatal condition**.
- Sunburn pain may be relieved with oatmeal baths or by adding baking soda to the bath water (one-half cup into cool or lukewarm water). See *Sunburn*, p. 161.
- A broken aloe vera leaf applied to the burned area may soothe the pain.
- While caring for your burn at home, be aware of signs of infection which can develop in 24 to 48 hours *(see Infected Wounds, p. 78).*

Second-degree burns

- Treat like first-degree burns if no bigger than two to three inches in diameter and not on face, hands, feet, groin, buttocks or a major joint — in which case you should **seek emergency care.**

Third-degree burns

- **Cover the burned area with a cool, damp, sterile dressing or clean cloth and seek emergency care immediately.**

Prevention

FOR ADULTS AND CHILDREN

- Conduct fire drills at home and work. Know the location of fire escapes when sleeping away from home.

- Install smoke detectors in every bedroom and on every floor and test them periodically.

- Keep emergency numbers by the telephone.

- Place a fire extinguisher in the kitchen and check the expiration date on a routine basis.

- Keep a large box of baking soda within easy reach of the stove.

- Keep a potted aloe vera plant in the kitchen (where most burns occur) to use the fresh jelly for treating minor burns.

- Never put lighter fluid on lit charcoal briquettes.

- Only use kerosene or other space heaters that have the UL (Underwriter's Laboratory) seal of approval.

- Always follow safety instructions when using chemicals, and note any warnings or precautions on container.

- Learn how to deal with an overheated engine, car fire, or live wire on a car.

- Never touch a downed electrical wire.

- Know where all electrical wiring is located before starting construction or renovation. This also applies to any kind of outdoor digging.

- Check with your utility company if you are unsure about the location of power lines in your area.

FOR CHILDREN

- Never leave a young child at home alone.
- Keep matches and chemicals out of reach.
- Turn pot handles toward the back of the stove while cooking.
- Never drink hot beverages with a child on your lap.
- Never place hot beverages or liquids near a table edge.
- Don't use mats or table cloths that can be pulled easily off a table.
- Make sure pajamas are flame-retardant.
- Cover electrical outlets when not in use.
- Set water heater thermostats no higher than 120° F to 125° F.

Final notes

FOR ALL TYPES AND DEGREES OF BURNS

- NEVER apply ointments, such as Vaseline, sprays, butter, oils or creams. They may slow healing and increase risk of infection. Use cool water instead.
- NEVER cover a burn with materials such as blankets, towels or tissue since fibers may become stuck to the wound. Use a clean sheet or sterile dressing.
- NEVER break blisters. Blisters protect the burn from infection and should only be ruptured if swelling constricts circulation.

Heat exhaustion

Too hot for comfort and safety

Heat exhaustion occurs when your body is not able to cool off and maintain a comfortable body temperature. Hot weather, excessive exercise and dehydration can cause the body to overheat. Small children and people who are frail, are older adults, are obese or have a chronic illness are at risk, as well as people in poor condition who overexert themselves.

Note your symptoms

- Headache
- Weakness
- Fatigue
- Dizziness
- Nausea
- Shallow breathing
- Muscle cramps

What you can do

If you are overheating:
- Move to a cooler place and remain quiet.
- Loosen clothing.
- If dizzy, lie down with head lower than feet.
- Drink small amounts of liquid frequently.
- Place cool, wet cloth on forehead.
- Watch for signs of shock and heat stroke (see *Shock*, p. 42).
- Do not consume alcohol or apply it to the skin.

Seek emergency help

Heat stroke is the critical stage of heat exhaustion and is a medical emergency. All of the body's cooling systems are overloaded when the body temperature reaches 104° F and continues to rise. Symptoms of heat stroke are:
- Hot, dry skin

1

- Bright red or flushed skin
- Body temperature of 105° F or greater
- Person becomes delirious, disoriented or unconscious

While waiting for help, sponge the victim's body with cool water or apply cool, wet sheets and monitor the victim's temperature every 10 minutes. Stop cooling if temperature drops suddenly or signs of shock develop with cool, clammy skin and weak, rapid pulse (see *Shock*, p. 42).

Call your doctor now

If symptoms are severe, become worse with self-care or last longer than one hour, seek professional medical care quickly.

Prevention

- Drink more than 10 eight-ounce glasses of water a day if exercising or working in hot weather.
- Stay in the shade or air-conditioned areas. Avoid sudden changes of temperature.
- Wear loose-fitting, light-colored clothing of natural fibers such as cotton or linen.
- Limit your activity and exercise during the hottest time of the day.
- Never leave an infant or child alone in a closed auto in hot weather.

Hypothermia and frostbite

When it's colder than you think

In *hypothermia* your body temperature drops below normal when body heat is lost faster than it can be produced. *Frostbite* is the freezing of the skin or tissue near the skin surface. These conditions can actually occur when the weather is windy or wet, yet still above freezing. Frail, inactive people, the elderly and small children are particularly susceptible.

Note your symptoms

HYPOTHERMIA

This condition can develop quickly and become a serious problem with little warning. Early symptoms include shivering, apathy, impaired judgment and cold, pale skin. As the body temperature continues to drop, shivering may stop; the abdomen and chest become cold, and there is slowing of the pulse and breathing. Weakness, drowsiness and confusion may quickly lead to unconsciousness.

FROSTBITE

Initially the skin feels soft to the touch but numb and tingly and may turn white. As the skin freezes and becomes hard, blisters may develop. In third-degree frostbite the skin may look blue or blotchy and the underlying tissue is hard and very cold.

What you can do

Treat for hypothermia before treating frostbite.

HYPOTHERMIA

- Get to warm, dry shelter.
- Rewarm slowly. Keep victim awake.
- Apply body heat from another person or warm, dry clothing or both.
- Give warm liquids and high-calorie food. **Do not give alcohol.**

1

What you can do

FROSTBITE

- Rewarm only if refreezing will not occur.
- Rewarm as quickly as possible.
- Warm small areas with breath or by placing them inside clothing and next to bare skin.
- Immerse body parts in warm (not hot) water of 104° F to 108° F for 15 to 20 minutes.
- Elevate and protect warmed part.
- Do not rub or massage frozen area — rubbing may cause further damage.
- Protect blisters. Do not break them.
- Aspirin or acetaminophen (Tylenol) may ease painful burning. **NEVER give aspirin to children/teenagers. It can cause Reye's syndrome, a rare but often fatal condition.**
- Watch for signs of infection (see *Infected Wounds*, p. 78).

Prevention

- Dress warmly in layers with wool and polypropylene for insulation and an outer layer that is windproof and waterproof.
- Wear a warm hat with ear protection. Wear mittens rather than gloves.
- Pace activities. Do not become exhausted or sweaty.
- Never touch cold metal with bare skin.
- Avoid alcohol and smoking before spending time in the cold.
- Eat well and carry extra food.
- Plan ahead and carry provisions in case of emergency or sudden weather changes.

Hypothermia and frostbite
DO THESE APPLY:

- **Unconsciousness**
- **Slowing in pulse and breathing**
- **Weakness, drowsiness or confusion**
- **Shivering stops and warming has not begun**

Until help arrives:

see *What You Can Do, Hypothermia,* p. 37

YES

SEEK
EMERGENCY
CARE

APPLY
EMERGENCY
FIRST AID

NO

- **Victim is small child, elderly or frail**
- **If you suspect frostbite:**
    - **Skin is hard, cold, white and blotchy or blue**
    - **Blisters develop**
- **Signs of infection 24 to 48 hours after frostbite:**
    - **Redness around the area or red streaks leading away**
    - **Swelling**
    - **Warmth or tenderness**
    - **Pus**
    - **Fever of 101° F or higher**
    - **Tender or swollen lymph nodes**

Until seen by doctor:

see *What You Can Do, Frostbite,* p. 38

YES

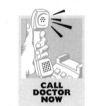

CALL
DOCTOR
NOW

Unconsciousness

To be out cold

When a person is unconscious, they are completely unaware of themselves and their surroundings. They have no control over body functions or movement. Usually they are not able to recall or remember any of the time spent in an unconscious state.

There are many causes of unconsciousness, including stroke, epilepsy, diabetic coma, head injury, alcohol intoxication, poisoning, heart attack, bleeding, electrocution and shock.

What you can do

IF SOMEONE HAS LOST CONSCIOUSNESS

- Check for breathing. If necessary, open the airway and begin rescue breathing (see *CPR*, p. 20 and *Choking*, p. 24).

- Check pulse. If no pulse, begin CPR (see *CPR*, p. 20).

- Call for emergency medical assistance.

- Keep the person warm unless you suspect heat stroke (see *Heat Exhaustion*, p. 35).

- Lay the person down face up, with their head below their heart level. Move them as little as possible and only to provide life support or safety. Do not move victim if you suspect a head or neck injury (see *Head/Spinal Injury*, p. 60).

- If there is vomit in the mouth, turn victim on their side to allow fluids to drain out.

- Look for medical identification or possible cause of unconsciousness.

- Do not give anything to eat or drink.

know
WHAT TO DO

Unconsciousness
DO THESE APPLY:

- **No response to shout or touch**
  Check breathing and pulse. Start CPR if necessary.
  see *CPR, pp. 20 - 23*
- **Vague response to shout and touch**
- **Loss of bladder and bowel control**
- **No recall of time and possible head injury**

YES

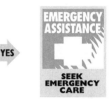

SEEK EMERGENCY CARE

APPLY EMERGENCY FIRST AID

NO

- **Awake and responsive after period of complete unconsciousness**

YES

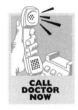

CALL DOCTOR NOW

1

Shock

Always an emergency

If your vital organs are unable to get the blood and oxygen they need, your body can go into shock. Many conditions can cause this urgent situation, including an injury, bleeding, pain, poisoning, extremely high or low body temperature, allergic reaction or a severe illness.

Shock is always an emergency and requires professional medical help immediately.

What you can do

PREPARING FOR AN EMERGENCY

- Learn your local emergency phone numbers. Post them somewhere handy.

- Wear identification to alert medical help if you have any allergies or chronic medical conditions.

WHEN YOU SEE SIGNS OF SHOCK

- Act immediately when you see any signs of shock. Do not wait to see if the victim improves on their own.

- Call your local emergency services number. Then, while you wait for help to arrive:

  - Have the victim lie down and elevate legs higher than heart, with support. **If head or neck injury is a possibility, keep victim flat and do not move them** (see *Head/Spinal Injury,* p. 60).

  - If victim vomits, roll them onto their side to allow fluid to drain out.

  - Control bleeding by applying direct pressure to wound (see *Control Severe Bleeding,* p. 47).

  - Keep victim warm unless cause of shock is heat stroke (see *Heat Exhaustion,* p. 35).

- Note the time. Take and record victim's pulse rate every five minutes. (Feel for the pulse of their heartbeat in wrist or side of neck with the tips of your index and middle fingers as shown on page 21, Figure 3. Count the number of beats in 15 seconds and multiply by four: 30 beats in 15 seconds x 4 = a pulse rate of 120 beats/minute.)

- Do not give anything to eat or drink.

- Comfort and reassure the victim while waiting for medical assistance.

- Look for evidence of cause, such as poison nearby (see *Poisoning*, p. 28) or medical-alert identification.

Shock

DO THESE APPLY:

- **Cool, pale, clammy skin**
- **Weak, rapid pulse**
- **Shallow, rapid breathing**
- **Confusion, anxiety or restlessness**
- **Faintness, weakness, dizziness or loss of consciousness**
- **Dilated pupils**
- **Nausea, vomiting or thirst**

see *What You Can Do*

YES

EMERGENCY ASSISTANCE

SEEK EMERGENCY CARE

APPLY EMERGENCY FIRST AID

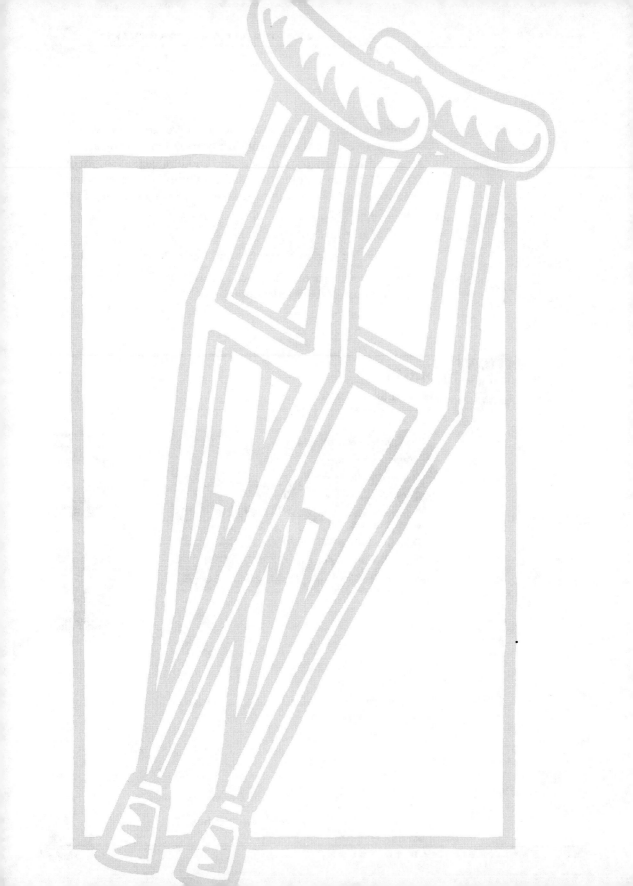

Injuries

2

WOUNDS

There are three kinds of wounds: cuts, abrasions and punctures. All of them — no matter how small — should be cared for quickly to promote healing, prevent infection and reduce scarring.

With every wound there is the potential for infection (for prevention and care of infected wounds, see *Infected Wounds,* p. 78). Get a routine tetanus booster every 10 years and keep up-to-date immunization records (see *Immunization Schedule,* p. 377). If you have a dirty wound and have not had a tetanus booster within the last five years, your doctor will probably recommend a booster injection.

Cuts

They need careful attention

There is rarely permanent damage from shallow, minor cuts (or *lacerations*) in which the wound is limited to the skin and the fatty tissue beneath it, and they usually can be treated easily at home.

In most minor cuts, bleeding is slow and stops on its own after a few minutes. Slightly deeper cuts can reach the veins, and cause steady blood flow that is slow and dark red. Pressure on the wound usually stops bleeding after a short period. The most serious type of external bleeding, however, is from a cut that strikes an artery. Bleeding is profuse and can be difficult to control even with pressure on the wound. Blood will be bright red and come in spurts as the heart beats. A person with severe bleeding can slip into shock (see *Shock,* p. 42, and *Control Severe Bleeding,* p. 47).

Stitches are usually not necessary if the edges of the cut can be pulled together with a bandage or sterile adhesive tape — except on the face, where scarring may be a problem. However, your doctor may *suture* (or stitch) cuts in areas subject to frequent movement, such as a finger; in young children, who would pull off bandages; or when a cut is more than one inch long, deep and with jagged edges. Suturing should take place within eight hours of injury for best results. Call your doctor if you're not sure whether you need stitches.

What you can do

CONTROL SEVERE BLEEDING

- Dial 911 or your local emergency services number. While waiting for help to arrive:

  - Have the injured person lie down with their head slightly lower than their body. Elevate their legs and the site of the bleeding.

  - Keep the victim warm to lessen the possibility of shock (see *Shock*, p. 42).

  - Remove large pieces of dirt and debris from the wound, but only if it can be done easily. DO NOT remove any impaled objects or try to clean the wound (see *Punctures*, p. 50).

  - Place a clean cloth over the wound and apply direct, steady pressure for 15 minutes. To avoid transmission of blood-borne infections, use your bare hands only if necessary.

  - DO NOT apply direct pressure if there is an object in the wound or a bone is protruding or visible. Apply pressure around the wound instead.

  - If the first cloth becomes soaked with blood, apply a fresh one over it while continuing steady pressure. Do not remove used bandages.

  - If bleeding does not slow or stop after 15 minutes, apply firm, continuous pressure on a pressure point between the wound and the heart to restrict blood flow through the major arteries. Pressure points are located on the inside upper arms and on the upper thighs in the groin area.

GIVE PROMPT ATTENTION TO MINOR WOUNDS

- Apply pressure on the wound for 10 or 15 minutes to stop bleeding, if necessary.
- Gently clean the cut with soap and water or 3% hydrogen peroxide, and a clean cloth. Be sure to remove dirt, glass and other particles. Antiseptic creams are not necessary and will not lessen the risk of infection or speed healing.
- Keep the cut uncovered and exposed to air if possible.
- If you must cover the cut, apply an antibiotic ointment to the wound and cover it with an adhesive bandage, perpendicular to the cut, so the edges are drawn together. Change the bandage once a day or when it gets wet.

WATCH FOR SIGNS OF INFECTION

Thorough cleansing of the wound is the best way to prevent infection and speed healing. Infection is more likely when a cut occurs in an area that is difficult to keep clean and dry, such as on a hand, foot or near a child's mouth. Signs of infection may begin about 24 to 48 hours after the injury. They include redness around the area or red streaks leading away, swelling, warmth or tenderness, pus, fever of 101° F or higher and tender or swollen lymph nodes (see *Infected Wounds*, p. 78).

Final notes

Deep cuts can sever or damage major blood vessels, nerves or tendons, so it is important to know the signs of a serious laceration. In general, be concerned more with cuts to the face, hands, chest, abdomen or back, which have the potential to be more critical than lacerations to other areas.

see *Know What To Do*, pp. 51 - 52

Abrasions

Routine events for most children

Scrapes, or *abrasions*, are routine in many families, especially those with young children. Scrapes from falls or other accidents scratch and tear the first few layers of skin. The injury is shallow but can be very painful because millions of nerve endings are exposed. The pain usually subsides within a few days as scabbing forms. These injuries are usually very dirty and must be cleaned thoroughly to prevent infection.

What you can do

- Clean the area with soap and warm water, making sure to remove all dirt and foreign particles.

- Leave skin flaps in place to act as a natural bandage. Dirty skin flaps can be cut away carefully with nail scissors. Stop cutting if it hurts.

- Place an ice pack over the wound for a few minutes to alleviate most of the pain. For protection, place a washcloth between bare skin and ice. Use a pain reliever such as aspirin, acetaminophen (Tylenol) or ibuprofen if mild pain persists. **NEVER give aspirin to children/ teenagers. It can cause Reye's syndrome, a rare but often fatal condition.**

- Watch for signs of infection (see *Infected Wounds*, p. 78).

Large scrapes can be treated with antibiotic ointment and covered with a sterile, nonstick bandage. Put the ointment on the bandage, rather than rubbing it on the scrape.

see *Know What To Do*, pp. 51 - 52

Punctures

Don't take them lightly

A puncture wound is a penetrating injury with a sharp-pointed object such as a nail. Seemingly minor puncture wounds sometimes can cause considerable internal damage and — because they can be hard to clean — can become easily infected. If you have not had a tetanus booster within the last five years, your doctor will probably recommend one to prevent *tetanus* (or "lockjaw").

What you can do

- **Seek emergency medical care if an object, such as a knife, projects from or is embedded in the skin**. Never try to pull the object out, since this could cause further injury. Very gently place a clean, damp cloth around the wound (for smaller objects, see *Splinters*, p. 67).

- Allow the wound to bleed freely to cleanse itself. Don't apply pressure unless blood is spurting out or is excessive (see *Control Severe Bleeding*, p. 47).

- If the puncture wound isn't serious enough to need emergency medical attention, wash it thoroughly with soap and water or hydrogen peroxide. Remove dirt carefully, using tweezers wiped with alcohol to extract debris. Pat wound dry with clean cloth and stop bleeding. Small wounds will stop bleeding on their own. For others, you may need to apply pressure with a gauze pad or clean cloth and elevate the area above the level of the heart.

- Antiseptics, such as mercurochrome and Merthiolate, aren't necessary and may cause pain. Nonprescription antibiotic ointments, such as Neosporin and Bacitracin, may help prevent infection. Apply them to the side of the bandage that touches the wound, rather than to the wound itself.

- Cover the wound with a sterile bandage. Change the dressing at least once a day and keep the area clean and dry.

- Remove bandage and soak the area in warm water a few times a day for four to five days to promote healing.

- Watch closely for signs of infection (see *Infected Wounds*, p. 78).

- Keep a well-stocked first-aid kit on hand (see *Home Pharmacy*, p. 364).

Final notes

Any wound that doesn't heal well in two weeks should be seen by a doctor. Infection is a common and potentially serious complication that can occur even with minor wounds (see *Infected Wounds*, p. 78). An infected wound will take longer to heal and is more likely to scar.

know WHAT TO DO

Cuts/abrasions/punctures
DO THESE APPLY:

- **Bleeding is steady or profuse, or in rhythmic spurts**
- **Wound continues to bleed through bandages even after 15 minutes of direct pressure and elevation**
- **Signs of shock are present: weakness; confusion; cold, pale, moist skin**

  see *Shock*, p. 42
- **Breathing is shallow and pulse is weak and rapid**
- **Wound involves head, chest, hand or abdomen, unless obviously minor**
- **Wound is deep and penetrates to muscle or bone**
- **An object, such as a knife, projects from or is embedded in wound**

  see *What You Can Do, Punctures*, p. 50

YES →

EMERGENCY ASSISTANCE

SEEK EMERGENCY CARE

NO

see next page

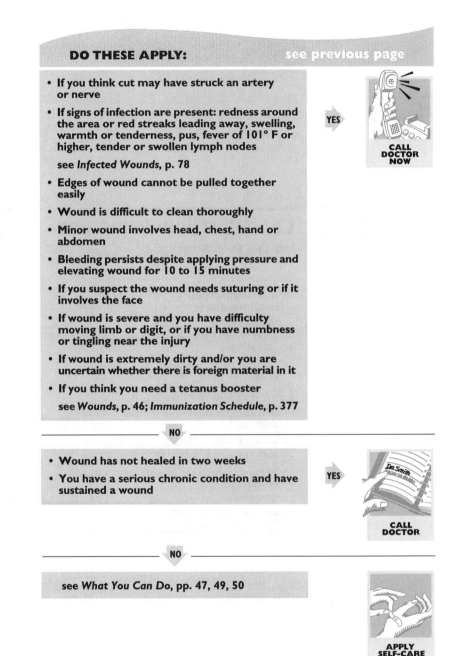

DO THESE APPLY:

see previous page

- If you think cut may have struck an artery or nerve
- If signs of infection are present: redness around the area or red streaks leading away, swelling, warmth or tenderness, pus, fever of 101° F or higher, tender or swollen lymph nodes

  see *Infected Wounds*, p. 78

- Edges of wound cannot be pulled together easily
- Wound is difficult to clean thoroughly
- Minor wound involves head, chest, hand or abdomen
- Bleeding persists despite applying pressure and elevating wound for 10 to 15 minutes
- If you suspect the wound needs suturing or if it involves the face
- If wound is severe and you have difficulty moving limb or digit, or if you have numbness or tingling near the injury
- If wound is extremely dirty and/or you are uncertain whether there is foreign material in it
- If you think you need a tetanus booster

  see *Wounds*, p. 46; *Immunization Schedule*, p. 377

YES

CALL DOCTOR NOW

NO

- Wound has not healed in two weeks
- You have a serious chronic condition and have sustained a wound

YES

CALL DOCTOR

NO

see *What You Can Do*, pp. 47, 49, 50

APPLY SELF-CARE

BITES/STINGS

If you have ever experienced an allergic reaction to any bite or sting, ask your doctor about wearing a medical-alert bracelet and getting a prescription for an anaphylactic kit. If you're planning outdoor activities such as camping, contact your local health department before you depart to get specific rabies information for the area where you'll be camping.

Animal/human bites

They can cause serious infections

The most common type of animal bites involve young children bitten by pets — usually dogs. In 5% of these cases, infection is common. (Cat bites become infected 30% to 50% of the time.) Adult human bites, which become infected in 15% to 20% of cases, most frequently result from injuries sustained in fist fights. Bites like these that break the skin can cause several types of serious infections:

- *Rabies*, most commonly from bites by dogs, cats, skunks, bats, raccoons, opossums, foxes and other wild animals

- *Tetanus*, which can develop after any kind of bite if you have not been inoculated within the last five years

- *Pasteurella* infection, commonly caused by cat bites

- Various bacteria or microorganisms can enter the wound and cause infection

What you can do

IMMEDIATELY AFTER BEING BITTEN

- Get emergency care if the bite seems serious, or affects the face or hands.

- Rinse and clean the wound immediately.

- Blood flow helps cleanse the wound. Control excessive bleeding by wrapping the wound with a bandage and applying direct pressure (see *Control Severe Bleeding*, p. 47).

- Watch for signs of infection, usually within 24 to 48 hours (see *Infected Wounds*, p. 78).

- Report all animal bites to the local health department, especially if the bite is from a wild animal or domestic animal whose rabies vaccination status is unknown. If a wild animal has symptoms of rabies (drooling, foaming at the mouth), it should be destroyed and tested. A domestic animal with uncertain rabies vaccination status should be observed for 15 days even if the animal appears healthy.

Prevention

- Treat all unfamiliar pets with caution.
- Don't try to touch any wild animal, especially if it appears sick.
- Obey "Beware of Dog" signs.
- Teach children not to touch or feed any animal they do not know — domestic or wild.
- Never leave an infant, young child or defenseless person unattended with a pet, especially a large dog.

see *Know What To Do*, p. 59

Insect bites/stings

Some little "critters" carry a big wallop

Most insect bites and stings are minor and the reaction is localized. Often an insect injects a substance with its bite that causes a painful, stinging sensation. More serious problems may arise if you're bitten by a poisonous insect — such as a black widow or brown recluse spider — or if you experience an allergic reaction.

What you can do

To know whether you need emergency care, see *Know What To Do*, p. 59.

IF EMERGENCY CARE IS REQUIRED

Until emergency care can be obtained:

- Apply ice or cold water to the bite for five minutes. For protection, place a washcloth between bare skin and ice.

- If the bite is on a hand or foot, keep the limb snugly bandaged above the bite for five minutes (but make sure there is still circulation to the limb). *Do not apply a tourniquet.*

- Keep the limb below the level of the heart.

WHEN EMERGENCY CARE IS NOT REQUIRED

- Scrape out or flick out any stinger that may be left in the skin by scraping it out with your fingernail. Avoid squeezing the stinger.

- Make a paste with water and baking soda or meat tenderizer and apply to painful area.

- Use calamine lotion or over-the-counter (OTC) hydrocortisone cream to reduce itching and inflammation.

- Apply ice. For protection, place a washcloth between bare skin and ice.

- If itching becomes severe, try an over-the-counter (OTC) oral antihistamine such as Benadryl or ChlorTrimeton.

Prevention

GENERAL PRECAUTIONS

- Avoid wearing perfume if you'll be spending time outdoors — it attracts bees.

- Get reliable instructions before trying to remove a beehive or nest. Follow directions on commercial products.

- If known to be allergic to bees, always carry an anaphylactic kit. You can get one with a prescription from your doctor.

see *Know What To Do,* p. 59

Snakebites

Most are not poisonous

More than 45,000 people are bitten by snakes each year, but only about 8,000 of those are by poisonous snakes. Fewer than 15 fatalities result from snakebites annually, and many of those occur because the bites are not treated.

DETERMINING IF THE SNAKE IS POISONOUS

Most venomous snakes in the United States (such as rattlesnakes, copperheads and water moccasins) are characterized by:

- Triangular-shaped head
- Elliptical-shaped (slit-like) eyes
- A depression (or pit) midway between the nostrils and eyes

Rattlesnakes produce a characteristic rattling sound with their tail. The water moccasin has a whitish, cottony lining in its mouth. The copperhead has a large, coppery head. Poisonous coral snakes have red, yellow and black rings along their body.

If you know, or suspect, the snake was poisonous, it is especially important to seek emergency medical care. If medical help is more than 30 or 40 minutes away, use a commercial snakebite kit within five minutes of the bite. Never use your mouth to suction the wound.

IF THE SNAKE IS NOT POISONOUS

Bites from nonpoisonous snakes generally are not harmful. If bitten by a snake you know is not poisonous:

- Rinse and clean the wound with soap and water.
- Don't try to stop the bleeding unless it is severe.
- Get a tetanus shot if you haven't had one in five or more years (see *Immunization Schedule*, p. 377).
- Watch for signs of infection (see *Infected Wounds*, p. 78).

2

What you can do

WHILE YOU WAIT FOR MEDICAL ATTENTION

- Lie down and try to remain calm. Stay as quiet as possible.
- Keep your body warm.
- Keep the bitten area lower than the level of the heart.
- Remove all jewelry near the affected area.
- Snugly wrap a bandage several inches above a bite on an arm or leg.
- Do not move the wounded area. Use a splint if possible.
- DO NOT take any drugs, including aspirin or alcohol. DO NOT apply heat or ice to the wound. DO NOT use a tourniquet. DO NOT cut into the wound to try to drain or suck out the venom.

know
WHAT
TO DO

Bites/stings

DO THESE APPLY:

- You experience symptoms of an allergic reaction following an insect bite: chest pain, palpitations or change in heart rate, difficulty breathing, violent coughing, loss of consciousness, fever of 101° F or higher, severe hives, tingling of mouth or throat, swelling of skin or lips, enlargement of stomach, intestinal spasms or cramping

- Severe pain or itching of wound, increased perspiration, weakness or listlessness, nausea, paralysis

- Bite by black widow or brown recluse spider, or other poisonous insect, marine animal or reptile

- Known sensitivity or allergy to insect causing bite

- Bite by a snake you think may be poisonous

- Any serious bite, especially if affecting face or hand

- Signs of infection within several hours of a cat bite: redness around the area or red streaks leading away, swelling, warmth or tenderness, pus, fever of 101° F or higher, tender or swollen lymph nodes

see *What You Can Do*, pp. 53, 55, 58

YES

EMERGENCY ASSISTANCE

SEEK EMERGENCY CARE

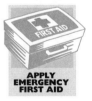

FIRST AID

APPLY EMERGENCY FIRST AID

NO

see next page

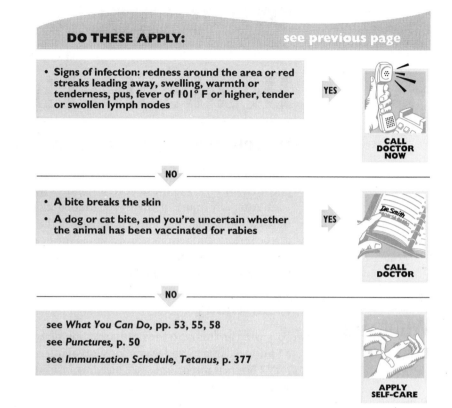

DO THESE APPLY: see previous page

- Signs of infection: redness around the area or red streaks leading away, swelling, warmth or tenderness, pus, fever of 101° F or higher, tender or swollen lymph nodes

YES ▶ CALL DOCTOR NOW

———————— NO ————————

- A bite breaks the skin
- A dog or cat bite, and you're uncertain whether the animal has been vaccinated for rabies

YES ▶ CALL DOCTOR

———————— NO ————————

see *What You Can Do,* pp. 53, 55, 58

see *Punctures,* p. 50

see *Immunization Schedule, Tetanus,* p. 377

APPLY SELF-CARE

OTHER INJURIES

Head/spinal injury

Watch closely, act quickly

Any trauma to the head or spine is cause for concern because of the potential for injury to the delicate structures within the brain and spinal cord. After any injury involving the head, neck or back it is important to watch for signs that may indicate damage to the brain or spinal cord. This can be serious and requires professional medical assistance immediately. Fortunately, most injuries are limited to the surrounding protective tissues and can be treated with self-care.

What you can do

HEAD INJURY

Following an injury to the head, treat any surface injury, protect from additional damage, and watch for signs of internal bleeding. Observation for 72 hours is important since bleeding inside the skull may be slow and symptoms may develop gradually.

- If there is external bleeding, apply pressure on the wound for 15 minutes or until bleeding stops completely. Use a clean cloth and if the blood soaks through, apply additional cloths over the first one.

- Apply ice or cold packs to ease pain and reduce swelling. A "goose egg" may develop. For protection, place a washcloth between bare skin and ice.

- Check for signs of bleeding inside the skull immediately after injury, then every two hours for the first 24 hours, every four hours for the next 24 hours, and every eight hours through the third day. Signs include:

  - **Changes in mental state** that may include unconsciousness, confusion, decrease in alertness, abnormally deep sleep, or difficulty waking up

- **Unequal size of pupils after the injury**; some people normally have a difference in pupil size, but a change after an injury can be a serious sign
- **Severe, forceful vomiting** that is repeated or continues (one single episode of vomiting may be a reaction to the pain)
- **Change or decrease in ability to move parts** of the body or a change in the ability to see, smell, hear, taste or touch
- Check for other injuries, especially to neck and back.
- Keep victim sitting or lying down with head slightly elevated to decrease swelling.
- Avoid heavy exercise or exertion for at least 72 hours.
- Be alert to chronic headache or changes in personality months after a head injury. These may be signs of very slow bleeding which can cause pressure on the brain much later.

2

SPINAL INJURY

Injury to the spine can occur in any accident involving the neck or back. Strain from incorrect positions or movement, and damage from disease such as arthritis can injure the spinal nerves. Self-care is directed toward preventing additional damage and permanent paralysis, decreasing symptoms and eliminating future injury.

What you can do

If you suspect a sudden injury to the spine:

- DO NOT MOVE THE PERSON unless there is an immediate threat to life, such as a fire.
- Call for professional medical help to move the victim. Keep the person still and warm. Do not give anything to eat or drink.
- If there is immediate danger and you must move the victim, **immobilize the neck and back**. Slide a board or other firm surface under the victim's head and back without moving the neck or back from the position it was in. Place soft, bulky material on each side of the head to prevent rotation.
- In a diving accident, **do not pull the victim from the water.** Float the person face up. The water will help support the neck and back.
- If there is much bleeding from the nose or mouth, roll the victim onto their side (the entire body needs to roll in one, even movement) without twisting the neck or back. If the bleeding is minor, wipe out the mouth and nose without moving the victim.

Prevention

- Wear your seat belt while in all motor vehicles and place children in proper car seats.
- Wear a helmet while biking, motorcycling, skating, skateboarding or horseback riding.
- Don't dive into shallow or unfamiliar water.
- Exercise to keep back, neck and abdominal muscles strong.

know
WHAT
TO DO

Head/spinal injury
DO THESE APPLY:

- Cessation of breathing or if no pulse; start CPR
  see *CPR, p. 20*
- Unconsciousness, confusion or any loss of memory
- Seizure or convulsions
- Bleeding from nose, ears, mouth or around eyes
- Clear fluid draining from nose
- Change in pupil size or sudden double vision
- Weakness, tingling or numbness in arms, legs or one side of body
- Loss of control of bladder or bowel
- Irregularity or slowing of breathing or heart rate

Do not move victim. Do not give anything to eat or drink.

see *What You Can Do, Head Injury, p. 60*

see *What You Can Do, Spinal Injury, p. 62*

YES

EMERGENCY ASSISTANCE
SEEK EMERGENCY CARE

FIRST AID
APPLY EMERGENCY FIRST AID

NO

- Continued or repeated vomiting
- Severe pain or headache
- Person under influence of drugs or alcohol
- A cut that may need stitches
- Victim under 2 years of age

Do not give anything to eat or drink.

see *What You Can Do, Head Injury, p. 60*

see *What You Can Do, Spinal Injury, p. 62*

YES

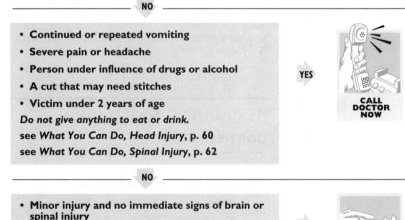
CALL DOCTOR NOW

NO

- Minor injury and no immediate signs of brain or spinal injury

see *What You Can Do, Head Injury, p. 60*

see *What You Can Do, Spinal Injury, p. 62*

YES

APPLY SELF-CARE

Accidental tooth loss

A real knockout

When a permanent tooth is knocked out, your dentist may be able to re-implant it successfully if the tooth tissue is kept alive. Your chances of saving a tooth are good up to one hour after injury. Baby teeth are not usually re-implanted since they eventually come out anyway.

What you can do

WHEN YOU INJURE OR LOSE A PERMANENT TOOTH

• Avoid touching the root end of the tooth.

• As long as the tooth is not contaminated or dirty, place it back in the gum socket.

• If unable to place in the socket, put tooth in cold, whole milk (not skim or powdered).

• Do not clean, wash or scrape the tooth. This may cause more damage.

Prevention

• Wear a protective dental guard or headgear when participating in sports.

• Know when and how to reach your dentist in an emergency.

 know WHAT TO DO

Accidental tooth loss

DO THESE APPLY:

• **Permanent tooth is knocked out**

• **No other signs of head or face injury**

see *What You Can Do*

Request emergency appointment for re-implantation by your dentist. Bring tooth with you.

• **Baby tooth is knocked out**

Request appointment to determine need for spacer.

YES ➤

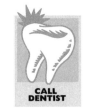

CALL DENTIST

Fishhooks

Hooking more than the fish

Fishhooks are designed with a barb to keep the fish hooked.
Unfortunately, the barb works the same way on people once the skin is
punctured. It is useful to know how to remove a fishhook for yourself or
a companion, especially if you are any distance from medical help. If the
injured person is a small child or unable to cooperate, a local anesthetic
to numb the injured area may be needed.

What you can do

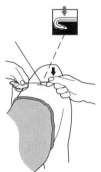

Figure 15

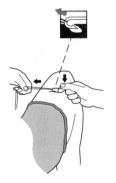

Figure 16

IF THE HOOK IS NEAR THE SKIN SURFACE

- **Step 1:** Apply ice or cold water to provide temporary numbing.
- **Step 2:** Loop a piece of fishing line through hook (Figure 15). Make the line long enough to grasp securely with your hand.
- **Step 3:** Grasp eye or shaft of hook with one hand and press down about one-eighth inch to disengage barb.
- **Step 4:** While still pressing down on hook, jerk the line parallel to skin surface so hook shaft leads barb out of skin (Figure 16).
- **Step 5:** Wash wound thoroughly with soap and water. Treat as you would a puncture wound (see *Punctures*, p. 50).

IF THE HOOK IS DEEPLY EMBEDDED

- **Step 1:** Apply ice or cold water to provide temporary numbing.
- **Step 2:** Push hook through the skin.
- **Step 3:** Cut off barb with wire cutters.
- **Step 4:** Pull hook back out.
- **Step 5:** Wash wound thoroughly with soap and water. Treat as you would a puncture wound (see *Punctures*, p. 50).

see *Know What To Do*, p. 66

Fishhooks

DO THESE APPLY:

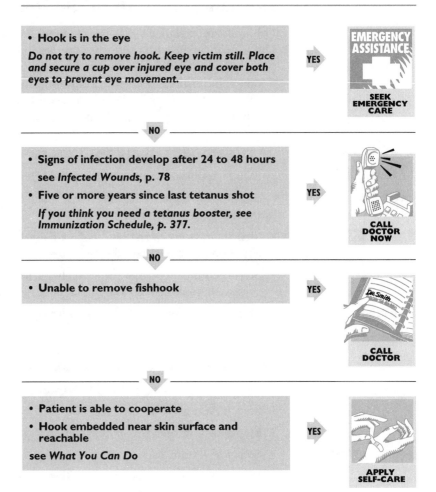

* **Hook is in the eye**

  Do not try to remove hook. Keep victim still. Place and secure a cup over injured eye and cover both eyes to prevent eye movement.

  YES → EMERGENCY ASSISTANCE — **SEEK EMERGENCY CARE**

NO

* **Signs of infection develop after 24 to 48 hours**

  see *Infected Wounds*, p. 78

* **Five or more years since last tetanus shot**

  If you think you need a tetanus booster, see Immunization Schedule, p. 377.

  YES → **CALL DOCTOR NOW**

NO

* **Unable to remove fishhook**

  YES → **CALL DOCTOR**

NO

* **Patient is able to cooperate**
* **Hook embedded near skin surface and reachable**

  see *What You Can Do*

  YES → **APPLY SELF-CARE**

Splinters

When you're stuck

A sharp, slender piece of wood, metal or glass can easily pierce the skin and become lodged. This type of injury usually can be treated at home by removing the splinter, cleaning the area and watching for signs of infection.

What you can do

IF THE SPLINTER CAN BE REACHED

- Grasp end of splinter with tweezers and gently pull it out along the entry track.
- Cleanse the area with soap and water.
- Keep area clean and dry; apply dry bandage if necessary.
- Watch for signs of infection:
    - Redness around the area or red streaks leading away
    - Swelling
    - Warmth and tenderness
    - Pus
    - Fever of 101° F or higher
    - Tender or swollen lymph nodes

IF THE SPLINTER IS DEEPLY EMBEDDED

- Clean a needle by dipping it in alcohol or holding it in a match flame.
- Pick the skin over end of splinter and make a small hole.
- Lift splinter with the tip of needle until it can be grasped by tweezers. Withdraw along the entry track.

see *Know What To Do*, p. 68

Splinters
DO THESE APPLY:

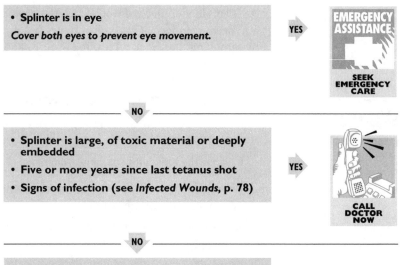

• **Splinter is in eye** *Cover both eyes to prevent eye movement.*	**YES**	**EMERGENCY ASSISTANCE** **SEEK EMERGENCY CARE**

NO

• **Splinter is large, of toxic material or deeply embedded** • **Five or more years since last tetanus shot** • **Signs of infection (see *Infected Wounds*, p. 78)**	**YES**	**CALL DOCTOR NOW**

NO

see *What You Can Do*

see *Immunization Schedule, Tetanus*, p. 377

see *Punctures*, p. 50

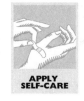

APPLY SELF-CARE

Smashed fingers

When you hit the wrong nail

Fingers often get smashed, pinched or jammed during daily activities. Most finger injuries are not serious. Although they may be quite painful and inconvenient, these injuries heal well with self-care at home. Serious injuries with possible bone fractures, severe bleeding or severed parts require professional medical help.

What you can do

- Immediately apply an ice pack or insert finger into ice-cold water to decrease the pain and reduce swelling. For protection, place a washcloth between bare skin and ice.

- Apply ice pack for 10 to 15 minutes every hour for two hours, then leave ice off for two hours. Repeat this cycle for 48 hours or until swelling is gone. Do not use heat as long as there is swelling.

- Remove any jewelry if you can do so without causing additional pain.

- If skin is broken, gently wash with soap, then dry. Apply soft, clean dressing.

- Splint and support injured finger by taping it to a nearby healthy one.

- Rest and elevate hand for 24 to 48 hours. Immobilize hand in a sling or use hand as little as possible.

- Take aspirin or ibuprofen to reduce swelling and pain. **NEVER give aspirin to children/teenagers. It can cause Reye's syndrome, a rare but often fatal condition.**

- When swelling is gone, apply warm compresses at intervals for comfort.

- Resume full range of motion as soon as swelling is gone. Gentle bending and movement will stretch the muscle tissue and prevent limited movement later.

- Stop any activity that causes pain to the finger.

DISLOCATED FINGERNAILS

- Trim the part of the nail that is still attached to avoid catching it on anything. It is not necessary to remove the nail.

- Keep area clean and watch for signs of infection (see *Infected Wounds*, p. 78).

- Protect the tip of the finger with a soft cloth or covering. A new nail will take one to two months to grow back.

BLOOD UNDER A NAIL

- Apply ice as soon as possible. For protection, place a washcloth between bare skin and ice.

- Make a hole in the nail to relieve pressure and pain:

  - Straighten a paper clip and hold it with a pair of pliers in a flame until it is red hot.

  - Place the tip of the paper clip on the nail and let it melt through. You need not push. A thick nail may take several tries. As soon as the hole is complete, blood will escape and the pain and pressure will ease.

- If the blood and pressure build up again, repeat the procedure using the same hole.

- Soak the finger three times a day for 15 minutes in a solution of equal parts water and hydrogen peroxide.

know
WHAT TO DO

Smashed fingers

DO THESE APPLY:

- **Finger is severed**

  Apply direct pressure with sterile bandage to control bleeding. Wrap severed part in clean or sterile gauze and place in plastic bag. Place bag on ice but do not let the tissue freeze. Bring the severed part with the injured person.

- **Severe bleeding or hemorrhage**

  Apply direct pressure with sterile bandage.

- **Finger deformed or bent into abnormal shape or bone protruding through skin**

  Immobilize the hand. Avoid unnecessary movement. Do not move or reposition finger.

- **Penetrating injury to finger**

  Do not attempt to remove object that is stuck in finger. Control bleeding and immobilize hand.

YES

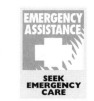

SEEK EMERGENCY CARE

APPLY EMERGENCY FIRST AID

NO

- **Numbness or a sensation of pins and needles in finger or hand**
- **A sensation of tearing or popping with movement**
- **Signs of infection (see *Infected Wounds*, p. 78)**
- **Movement painful for 24 hours or more**
- **Unable to remove jewelry due to swelling**
- **Torn skin that is dirty and it has been five or more years since last tetanus shot**

YES

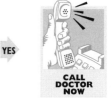

CALL DOCTOR NOW

NO

- **Torn skin that is clean and it has been 10 or more years since last tetanus shot**

  see *Immunization Schedule, Tetanus*, p. 377

- **Pain and swelling do not ease with self-care**

YES

CALL DOCTOR

NO

see *What You Can Do*

APPLY SELF-CARE

Strains and sprains

Muscle wear and tear

A strain is an injury to a muscle caused by over-stretching. Also called a "pulled muscle," the elastic fibers that make up the muscle are overextended and may tear, bleed and contract.

A sprain is an injury to a ligament and other soft tissue around a joint. Ligaments are bands of fiber that connect the bones at a joint. They can be stretched or torn when a joint is twisted, "jammed" or overextended. With a sprain, slight bleeding may produce skin discoloration which resolves slowly.

What you can do

The basic treatment for strains and sprains is a two-part process: **RICE** (rest, ice, compression, elevation) to treat the immediate injury and **MSA** (movement, strength, alternate activity) to help the injury heal and prevent further problems.

Begin the **RICE** process **immediately** following the injury:

- **Rest.** Do not put weight on injured joint or muscle, and limit movement in the area of the injury. Use crutches, splints or a sling as needed.

- **Ice.** Apply ice pack for 10 to 15 minutes every hour for two hours, then leave ice off for two hours. Repeat this cycle for 48 hours or until swelling is gone. For protection, place a washcloth between bare skin and ice. Do not use heat as long as there is swelling.

- **Compress.** Wrap injured area in an elastic bandage for support and protection.

- **Elevate.** Place injured part on pillows while you apply ice and anytime you are seated or lying down. Raise injured area above the level of your heart whenever possible.

Aspirin and ibuprofen may ease pain and inflammation. Acetaminophen (Tylenol) eases discomfort but does not decrease inflammation. Do not use other drugs to mask pain in order to continue using the injured part. **NEVER give aspirin to children/teenagers. It can cause Reye's syndrome, a rare but often fatal condition.**

The **MSA** process can be started only if the initial swelling is gone:

- **Movement**. Begin gently moving the joint to resume full range of motion.

- **Strength**. After the swelling is gone and a full range of motion is reached, gradually begin to strengthen the injured part. Slow, gentle stretching during the healing process will make scar tissue flexible and prevent limited movement later.

- **Alternate activities**. Resume regular exercise through activities and sports that do not place a strain on the injured area. Go slowly and stop any activity that causes discomfort.

Any increase in pain or return of swelling is a sign to stop **MSA** and resume **RICE**.

Prevention

- Use correct form in all work and play activities.
- Adjust equipment and furniture to fit your needs.
- Go slowly when starting a new activity or sport.
- Use warm-up and cool-down exercises to help your body prepare and recover safely.
- Take frequent breaks when performing any continuous activity.
- Do not push beyond your strength or ability; advance your skill level gradually.

see *Know What To Do*, p. 74

Strains and sprains
DO THESE APPLY:

After an injury there is:

- **Excruciating pain**
- **Obvious deformity of an extremity or suspicion of a fracture**
- **Tearing or popping sensation in the knee**

Splint or support injured area to keep it immobile (see What You Can Do, p. 76). Do not attempt to straighten injured part. Apply ice pack immediately. For protection, place a washcloth between bare skin and ice.

see *Broken Bones,* p. 75

see *Knee Pain,* p. 287

YES

SEEK EMERGENCY CARE

NO

- **Injured area is greatly swollen, discolored, unstable**

Splint or support injured area to keep it immobile (see What You Can Do, p. 76). Do not attempt to straighten injured part. Apply ice pack immediately. For protection, place a washcloth between bare skin and ice.

YES

CALL DOCTOR NOW

NO

- **No decrease in pain or swelling after two or three days of self-care with RICE**

see *What You Can Do*

Continue RICE until appointment.

YES

CALL DOCTOR

NO

- **Pain or swelling in joint or muscle following a related activity or movement**

  Start RICE immediately.

  see *What You Can Do*

- **Pain is decreasing and swelling is going away with RICE**

  Continue until swelling is gone and then start MSA. Full healing may take four or more weeks.

YES

APPLY SELF-CARE

Broken bones

When in doubt, splint

It is often difficult to tell if a bone has been broken or *fractured* in an injury. Unless the fracture is obvious, an x-ray may be needed to be sure.

The break may be a small crack such as a *stress fracture* caused by overuse or *greenstick fracture* often found in children, a *simple fracture* with the bone ends separated but in alignment, or a *compound fracture* where the soft tissue in the area is torn and the bone protrudes through the skin.

Although the treatment is similar for all fractures, the seriousness varies depending on which bone is broken, the type of break and if there are other associated injuries.

SUSPECT A FRACTURE IF

• Injured part is bent or deformed

• Bone is poking through the skin

• There is a bump or irregularity along the bone

• A cracking or snapping sound was heard at the time of injury

• There is rapid swelling or bruising immediately after the injury

2

What you can do

- Assume there may be a fracture.

- Immobilize and support the injured area with a splint. To splint, attach a stiff object (such as a rolled-up magazine or newspaper or a cane) to the injured limb with a rope or belt. Position the splint so the injured limb cannot bend.

- To immobilize and support a possible fractured toe, gently tape it to an adjacent toe.

- Do not attempt to move an abnormally bent or displaced bone back into place. Splint it as it is. Apply ice pack for 10 to 15 minutes every hour for two hours, then leave ice off for two hours. Repeat this cycle for 48 hours or until swelling is gone. For protection, place a washcloth between bare skin and ice. Do not use heat so long as there is swelling.

- Wrap the injury with an elastic bandage to immobilize and compress the area. Loosen the bandage if it becomes too tight.

- Elevate injured area.

- Avoid any unnecessary movement. Rest injury for at least 24 to 48 hours.

Use aspirin or ibuprofen to ease pain and inflammation. **NEVER give aspirin to children/teenagers. It can cause Reye's syndrome, a rare but often fatal condition.**

know
WHAT
TO DO

Broken bones
DO THESE APPLY:

- Limb is cold, blue or numb
- Injury is to pelvis or thigh
- Signs of shock (cool, clammy, pale skin; dizziness or light-headedness; thirst)

  Keep victim lying down and covered to stay warm. Do not give anything to eat or drink.

- Shortness of breath or difficulty breathing after chest injury

  Keep victim quiet. Place in sitting position to assist breathing.

- Bone protruding through skin
- Suspect fracture near a joint
- Injured part is crooked or deformed
- Heavy bleeding or blood spurting out

  Cover open wound with clean, dry cloth. Apply direct pressure on bleeding wound with a sterile or clean cloth. Apply only enough pressure to stop bleeding. If blood soaks through, apply another bandage. Do not remove first one. Do not apply tourniquet.

YES ▶

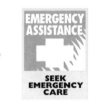
EMERGENCY ASSISTANCE
SEEK EMERGENCY CARE

FIRST AID
APPLY EMERGENCY FIRST AID

— **NO** —

- Injured part is unstable or unable to bear weight
- Large amount of swelling or bruising immediately after injury

see *What You Can Do*

YES ▶

CALL DOCTOR NOW

— **NO** —

- Injured area does not improve after 48 hours of self-care

YES ▶

Dr. Smith
CALL DOCTOR

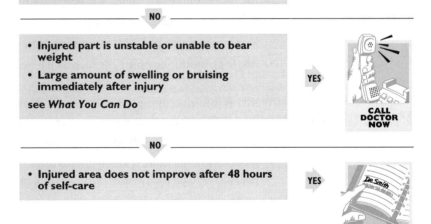

Infected wounds

Care can prevent infection

Any wound can become infected, particularly if it has not been thoroughly cleaned. An infected wound will take longer to heal, is more likely to scar and can result in serious complications, including death. Take the treatment of any wound seriously, and be alert for signs of infection.

Note your symptoms

Signs of an infected wound include:

- Redness around the area or red streaks leading away
- Swelling
- Warmth and tenderness
- Pus
- Fever of 101° F or higher
- Tender or swollen lymph nodes

What you can do

With your doctor's approval:

- Expose wound to air unless it is necessary to bandage it.
- Use a sterile bandage and change it daily or if it becomes wet.
- Remove bandage and soak wound in warm water several times a day.
- Apply an antibiotic ointment such as Bacitracin or Neosporin.

Prevention

Ward off infection by taking some simple steps as soon as the injury occurs. If the wound does not require emergency care:

- Clean it thoroughly with mild soap and warm water.
- Remove foreign objects and large particles of dirt with tweezers if necessary. Wipe the tweezers with alcohol first to disinfect them.
- Avoid using antiseptics, which can damage skin tissue.

- Keep your tetanus immunization up to date. You should get a routine tetanus booster every 10 years. However, if you have a dirty wound and have not had a booster within the last five years, your doctor may recommend a booster injection.

Final notes

Symptoms of infection generally begin to appear about 24 to 48 hours after the injury, although the potential for infection continues until healing is complete. People with diabetes and patients with organ transplants or cancer are at higher risk of infection.

know WHAT TO DO

Infected wounds

DO THESE APPLY:

- **Signs of infection develop:**
  - **Redness around the area or red streaks leading away**
  - **Swelling**
  - **Warmth or tenderness**
  - **Pus**
  - **Fever of 101° F or higher**
  - **Tender or swollen lymph nodes**
- **Wound has not healed well within two weeks**

YES

CALL DOCTOR NOW

— NO —

see *What You Can Do*
see *Wounds*, p. 46

APPLY SELF-CARE

Infant/child

CHILDHOOD RASHES

Baby rashes

Common but not harmful

The bumps and splotches on a new baby may be worrisome to a parent, but they aren't usually harmful. The following are the most common infant rashes. Only diaper rash and prickly heat rash require any treatment.

CHILDHOOD RASHES

Type	Symptoms	Self-Care
Acne	Acne on forehead, cheeks and chin, beginning at 2 to 4 weeks old	Wash face daily with cloth, water and mild soap; usually clears up spontaneously in six months to one year
Cradle Cap	Thick yellow crust on scalp and/or behind ears; face and scalp can also look red and inflamed; no fever; in severe cases yellowish-red pimples are seen along hairline, ears, eyebrows, nose and throat	Use mild baby shampoo daily; apply warm mineral oil to scalp 10 minutes before shampooing to loosen scales; gently comb; cradle cap tends to recur
Diaper Rash	Redness in diaper area. If redness extends beyond diaper area with small red spots or blisters, this can indicate a yeast or bacterial infection; call doctor now	Change diaper frequently; wash skin with soap and water, dry well; avoid disposable diapers, plastic pants until healed; Desitin or A&D ointment help protect the skin and promote healing
Erythema Toxicum	Flat, red splotches on arms, legs, chest, back and face, appearing before 5 days old	No treatment needed
Milia	Small white bumps on forehead, nose and cheeks	No treatment needed
Prickly Heat (Sweat) Rash	Small, red bumps in skin folds, especially on head, neck and shoulders	Dress baby lightly, provide less-humid environment; avoid ointments or creams that block pores

If rash is accompanied by fever or general malaise, consult your doctor (see *Fever*, p. 112).

CHILDHOOD DISEASES

Chicken pox

A common childhood disease

Chicken pox (or *varicella*) is a common, highly contagious viral disease most likely to occur in children ages 2 to 10. For adults it's relatively uncommon but can create serious complications when contracted, especially for pregnant women and their unborn child.

Chicken pox is contagious for about a week, from 24 to 36 hours before the rash appears until all the pox sores are scabbed over. Upon exposure, it takes an average of 14 to 16 days for symptoms to develop. Having chicken pox once usually gives lifelong immunity against the disease.

After you've had chicken pox, the virus takes up residence in a bundle of sensory nerve cells connected to the spinal cord. For most people the virus remains dormant. However, in some cases the virus is reactivated and travels down the nerve infecting the surrounding skin with a rash that turns into blisters. This is called *shingles*. No one knows for sure what reactivates the virus, but stress, trauma and certain illnesses can be triggers. Shingles usually occurs on one side of the body (most often on the torso) and is accompanied by sharp nerve pain. Acyclovir is often prescribed to lessen symptoms.

If you have shingles, it is possible to pass chicken pox on to someone who has never had the disease, although the virus is not often spread this way. Call your CareWise Nurse if you would like more information.

Note the symptoms

Early signs include a vague feeling of discomfort, mild headache, a cough and a low-grade fever. The rash appears as red bumps with tiny fluid-filled blisters. The blisters crust over within six to eight hours. For five or six days, the rash will appear on various sites of the body, and can include the mucous membranes of the eyes, mouth and vagina. The rash is extremely itchy and can cause permanent scars (slight, round depressions in the skin), especially if the scabs are scratched off. The scabs are present

3

even after chicken pox is no longer contagious. Usually people start to feel better before they look better.

Chicken pox is usually mild in healthy children, but can be more serious in adults or those with immune-system disorders.

Complications from chicken pox include an infected pox, pneumonia and, on rare occasions, *encephalitis* (an inflammation of the brain).

Chicken pox is very serious in newborns. If a mother has chicken pox four days or less before delivery, there is a 20% chance that the infant will be born with the disease. This is fatal for the infant in up to 30% of the cases.

Prevention

A new vaccine called *Varivax* (and referred to as the VZV vaccination) has been approved for use in the U.S. The American Academy of Pediatrics recommends including VZV as part of a child's immunization program (see *Immunization Schedule*, p. 377). The recommended dosage is:

- One dose given to infants between the age of 12-18 months
- Two doses given four to eight weeks apart to teens and adults who have never had chicken pox

Immunity from the chicken pox vaccine is expected to last about nine years.

What you can do

Treatment for chicken pox is directed toward relieving symptoms and watching for complications. Apply cool, wet compresses. Take an oatmeal bath (one-half to one cup of oatmeal in a tub of lukewarm water). Apply calamine lotion with a cotton swab to the itchy areas, except the mucous membranes (such as the mouth, eyes or vagina). Adults can take an antihistamine, but a pediatrician should be consulted about use in young children. Use mitts on infants and very young children, to avoid scratching.

Acetaminophen (Tylenol) will reduce fever. **NEVER give aspirin to children/teenagers. It can cause Reye's syndrome, a rare but often fatal condition. Children with chicken pox are at increased risk for Reye's syndrome.** If necessary, talk with your doctor about chicken pox over the telephone instead of taking your child into the office. This eliminates the risk of exposing others to the disease.

Chicken pox
DO THESE APPLY:

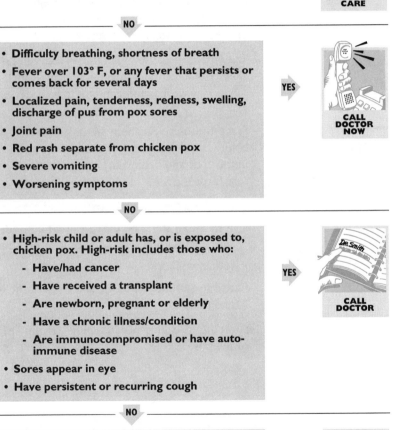

- Significant respiratory distress — such as rapid breathing or difficulty breathing and/or bluish discoloration to the skin
- Altered mental state or severe headache

YES → **EMERGENCY ASSISTANCE**

SEEK EMERGENCY CARE

— NO —

- Difficulty breathing, shortness of breath
- Fever over 103° F, or any fever that persists or comes back for several days
- Localized pain, tenderness, redness, swelling, discharge of pus from pox sores
- Joint pain
- Red rash separate from chicken pox
- Severe vomiting
- Worsening symptoms

YES →

CALL DOCTOR NOW

— NO —

- High-risk child or adult has, or is exposed to, chicken pox. High-risk includes those who:
    - Have/had cancer
    - Have received a transplant
    - Are newborn, pregnant or elderly
    - Have a chronic illness/condition
    - Are immunocompromised or have auto-immune disease
- Sores appear in eye
- Have persistent or recurring cough

YES →

CALL DOCTOR

— NO —

see *What You Can Do*

APPLY SELF-CARE

3

Rubella

Immunization is the best medicine

Rubella, also known as *German measles* and three-day measles, is a mild virus characterized by a flat or slightly raised pink or red rash.

The greatest danger is to pregnant women, who may pass on *congenital rubella syndrome* to their unborn child. This can result in birth defects — or even death — for the baby. If a pregnant woman contracts rubella during the first trimester of pregnancy, there is a chance that the fetus will develop abnormally in some way.

The virus is usually spread through coughing and sneezing, or through close contact with an infected person. Rubella can be transmitted to others one week before, and up to four days after, the onset of the rash.

Note the symptoms

Symptoms develop about 16 days after exposure. About five to 10 days before the rash appears, you may have swollen and tender lymph glands in the neck and behind the ears, mild fever, malaise, sneezing and a sore throat.

Other characteristic symptoms include:

* A rash that starts on the face and forehead, spreading quickly to the torso, arms and legs, and lasting about one day in each area
* A flushed face
* Redness of the *soft palate* (the back of the roof of the mouth) and throat

Some adults experience headache, joint pain, weariness and a stuffy and runny nose.

Prevention

Immunization is the safest and most effective way of preventing rubella. The vaccine is usually given in combination with those for measles and mumps in the *MMR* vaccine. All babies around 12 months old should be immunized, followed by another immunization by age 4 to 6 years (where required by health authorities for school entry; otherwise given at 11 to 12 years old — check with your doctor). For more information see *Immunization Schedule*, p. 377.

Women should make sure they are not pregnant before receiving the rubella vaccine, then diligently practice a reliable form of birth control for at least three months after the immunization. Some women might experience mild joint pain following the vaccination.

What you can do

To avoid spreading the infection and speed recuperation:

- Stay at home until the rash and swelling subside or as recommended by your doctor.

- If fever rises above 101° F, drink plenty of fluids. Sponge the face and upper body with lukewarm water.

- Acetaminophen (Tylenol) or anti-inflammatories may provide comfort. **NEVER give aspirin to children/teenagers. It can cause Reye's syndrome, a rare but often fatal condition**.

see *Know What To Do*, p. 88

3

Rubella

DO THESE APPLY:

- You have rubella and experience extreme drowsiness, headaches, sensitivity to bright light, or convulsions (suspect *encephalitis*, a brain inflammation and a very serious complication)

YES → **EMERGENCY ASSISTANCE**

SEEK EMERGENCY CARE

— **NO** —

- You have rubella and develop ear pain (suspect *otitis media*, a middle ear infection, see p. 103)
- You suspect rubella and are in the first trimester of pregnancy

YES → **CALL DOCTOR NOW**

— **NO** —

- You suspect rubella

YES → **CALL DOCTOR**

— **NO** —

see *What You Can Do*

APPLY SELF-CARE

Measles

Very common and contagious

Measles, also known as *rubeola* or red measles, is one of the most common and contagious diseases in the world. Although a person of any age can be affected, measles occurs most often in children, killing one million young people worldwide every year.

Widespread immunization programs in the mid-1960s began a sharp decline in the number of children affected. However, new trends have been observed in the United States recently, with outbreaks occurring in preschool-aged children who have not been immunized, as well as in previously immunized teenagers and young adults.

The virus is extremely contagious and is spread by coughing and sneezing. An infected person can infect others from two to four days before the rash appears — the most contagious period — and up to about five days after. Once individuals have been infected, they are usually immune to the disease for the rest of their lives. An infant usually is protected for the first year of life because of antibodies it has received from its mother.

Note the symptoms

Symptoms develop seven to 14 days after exposure to the virus and can include fever, sneezing, sore throat, persistent coughing and malaise. There may be eye irritation with redness, swelling and discharge.

Two to four days later, tiny red spots — with centers that look like grains of white sand or salt — appear on the insides of the cheeks by the upper back molars, and sometimes on the eyes and vaginal area. They last one to four days. You may also have a red throat, yellowish coating on the tonsils and swollen glands.

A brick-red, blotchy rash typically appears one to two days after the spots in the mouth appear. The rash starts on the face and behind the ears, spreading to the torso and extremities. It fades in the same order it appears. Often there is mild itching.

At the peak of illness, you may develop a fever of 104° F or higher, swelling around the mouth, a hacking cough and sensitivity to bright light. The fever should fall and the rash start to fade about three to five days after it appears. It may leave a coppery-brown discoloration and some scaliness, which will gradually fade. Measles usually lasts 10 to 14 days.

Prevention

Vaccination for measles is the key to prevention. The live virus vaccine is usually given in combination with mumps and rubella (*MMR*) vaccines. It is very safe, although a small number of people develop a high fever (over 101° F) five to 12 days after the injection. This is sometimes followed by a rash.

All babies around 12 months old should be immunized, followed by another immunization by age 4 to 6 years (where required by health authorities for school entry; otherwise given at 11 to 12 years old — check with your doctor). For more information see *Immunization Schedule*, p. 377.

People who have not been vaccinated and are exposed to measles may be protected if they are given the live vaccine within two days of exposure. The illness also may be averted by a measles immune globulin or immune serum globulin shot given immediately after exposure. (These injections are of no use once symptoms appear.)

What you can do

- Stay at home for a week after the rash disappears to avoid infecting others.

- Rest in bed (a darkened room may be most comfortable) until the fever disappears. However, it is not necessary to force bed rest on a child who is happy playing quietly.

- If the fever rises above 100.5° F, sponge the face and upper body with lukewarm water.

- Drink plenty of fluids.

- Try cough medicine to relieve cough symptoms.

- Take pain relievers for headache, fever and general discomfort. **NEVER give aspirin to children/teenagers. It can cause Reye's syndrome, a rare but often fatal condition.** Acetaminophen (Tylenol) is a safe alternative.

- Avoid exposure to individuals with streptococcal infections.

Final notes

Most people experience a smooth recovery from measles, but complications can develop. They include respiratory tract diseases such as pneumonia, bronchitis and croup; and bacterial infections in the eyes, lungs, ears and other areas (refer to index for more on these topics). *Encephalitis* (an infection in the brain) is a rare but life-threatening complication.

Measles

DO THESE APPLY:

- Measles with severe lethargy, headache, vomiting or convulsions
- Measles with bleeding from nose, mouth or rectum, or bleeding under the skin
- Measles with signs of pneumonia, such as difficulty breathing, or blue or gray color to lips or under nails

YES →

EMERGENCY ASSISTANCE

SEEK EMERGENCY CARE

NO

- You have measles and develop earache, rapid breathing or sore throat
- You suspect measles

YES →

CALL DOCTOR

NO

see *What You Can Do*

APPLY SELF-CARE

Mumps

Prevention is the best medicine

Mumps is a viral disease that usually causes painful swelling of the salivary glands. The virus is spread through coughing or sneezing or direct contact with saliva-contaminated materials. Infected persons can transmit the disease six or seven days before symptoms develop and up to nine days after. Once a person has had mumps or been vaccinated, they are usually immune for life.

Note the symptoms

Almost one-third of those infected do not develop symptoms. Others will start noticing symptoms 14 to 21 days after being exposed. Symptoms may include chills, headache, loss of appetite, malaise or a low- to moderate-grade fever.

The salivary glands between the ear and the angle of the jaw (the *parotids*) typically swell and become tender, as does the face. The combination creates the chipmunk-cheek look. The first sign of swelling may be pain while chewing or swallowing, especially when consuming anything acidic, like pickles or lemon juice.

A fever of 103° F to 104° F is common in adults but not typical in young children. Symptoms usually last two weeks or less.

Prevention

Mumps live virus vaccine is the answer to preventing mumps. This vaccine is safe and highly effective, and is usually combined with vaccines for measles and rubella in the *MMR* vaccine (see *Immunization Schedule*, p. 377).

All babies around 12 months old should be immunized, followed by another immunization by age 4 to 6 years (where required by health authorities for school entry; otherwise given at 11 to 12 years old — check with your doctor). Babies up to 1 year old are usually immune because they still carry antibodies from their mother. The vaccine shouldn't be given to pregnant women or those with weakened immune systems.

What you can do

To speed recuperation and avoid spreading the infection:

- Stay home until the swelling goes down or your doctor recommends returning to work or school.

- Bed rest is helpful until the fever subsides, but shouldn't be forced on a child who is happy playing quietly.

- Drink plenty of fluids but avoid acidic ones like orange juice.

- Take pain relievers for headache and general discomfort.

- **NEVER give aspirin to children/teenagers. It can cause Reye's syndrome, a rare but often fatal condition.** Acetaminophen (Tylenol) is a safe alternative.

Final notes

Complications of mumps, though rare in an otherwise healthy individual, are more common in adults than in children. These complications include an inflammation of the testes (*orchitis*) in males past puberty; an inflammation of the ovaries (*oophoritis*) in females past puberty; an inflammation of the membranes of the brain or spinal cord (*meningitis*) (see *Meningitis*, p. 271); and an inflammation of the pancreas (*pancreatitis*).

see *Know What To Do*, p. 94

3

Mumps

DO THESE APPLY:

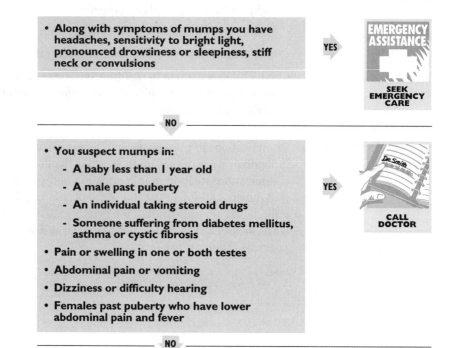

- Along with symptoms of mumps you have headaches, sensitivity to bright light, pronounced drowsiness or sleepiness, stiff neck or convulsions

YES → **EMERGENCY ASSISTANCE**

SEEK EMERGENCY CARE

NO

- You suspect mumps in:
    - A baby less than 1 year old
    - A male past puberty
    - An individual taking steroid drugs
    - Someone suffering from diabetes mellitus, asthma or cystic fibrosis
- Pain or swelling in one or both testes
- Abdominal pain or vomiting
- Dizziness or difficulty hearing
- Females past puberty who have lower abdominal pain and fever

YES → **CALL DOCTOR**

NO

see *What You Can Do*

APPLY SELF-CARE

Roseola

A harmless childhood virus

Roseola is a virus that mainly affects children between the ages of 6 months and 3 years, causing a rash and high fever. These symptoms are usually more alarming to parents than they are threatening to a young child's health. It's unclear how the virus is transmitted, but once children have had it, they won't get it again.

Note the symptoms

Roseola has a seven- to 17-day incubation period. Symptoms may include:

- Fever and irritability which occur suddenly. The fever may be as high as 105° F, and last three to five days. Even with this high fever, a child may remain alert and active.

- A mild sore throat

- Slight swelling of the lymph glands in the neck and behind the ears

- On the fourth or fifth day, temperatures often drop suddenly to normal or below.

- As the temperature falls, a mild rash usually appears on the torso and may extend to the neck, arms or thighs. These pink, well-defined patches will turn white when touched with light pressure and may be slightly bumpy. The rash may last from a few hours to a few days and may be so mild that it goes unnoticed.

The sudden high fever of roseola may cause a seizure (see *Fever*, p. 112). Although frightening, febrile seizures seldom cause problems. However, it is essential to treat the fever promptly (see below).

What you can do

There is no medication for treating roseola, but you can make your child more comfortable by:

- Attempting to relieve a high fever with sponge baths (swab the child's neck and upper body with lukewarm water)

- Keeping a fever down with acetaminophen (Tylenol); use as directed. **NEVER give children/teenagers aspirin. It can cause Reye's syndrome, a rare but often fatal condition.**

3

Roseola

DO THESE APPLY:

• **Seizures or severe lethargy**

YES → **CALL DOCTOR NOW**

NO

• **Fever of 103° F or higher in a child less than 2 years old that does not respond to self-care**
• **You suspect roseola**

YES → **CALL DOCTOR**

NO

see *What You Can Do*

APPLY SELF-CARE

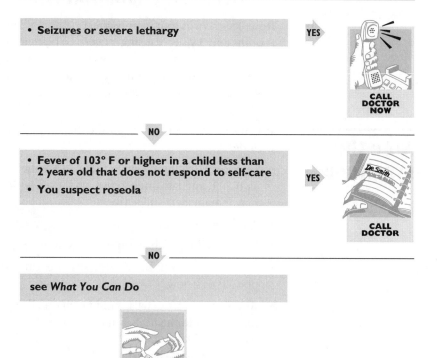

DIFFERENT SYMPTOMS?

see *Skin Symptoms,* p. 127

see *Fever,* p. 112

Scarlet fever

Strep throat with a rash

Scarlet fever is caused by a streptococcal infection, usually of the throat (see *Sore Throat*, p. 174) and gets its name from its characteristic red rash.

It is highly contagious, so all members of a household should be tested for the infection if one member is found to have it. It requires a trip to the doctor for a throat culture and to get antibiotics.

Note the symptoms

- A high fever is sometimes accompanied by a headache or stomachache, vomiting and/or a sore throat.

- The rash is red and fine, sometimes described as feeling like sandpaper. It appears 12 to 48 hours after the illness begins and within 24 hours often covers the entire body. It is most prominent on the cheeks, chest, abdomen and groin. The area around the mouth is pale. Little bumps on the tongue get progressively bigger and redder, until the tongue looks like it's coated with strawberries. It may become swollen. Glands in the neck may also become swollen.

- After the rash subsides, the skin may peel for several weeks, especially on the palms of the hands.

Final notes

Antibiotics are particularly important in treating scarlet fever because they can prevent *rheumatic fever*, a complication caused by the streptococcal infection which can result in heart damage.

see *Know What To Do*, p. 98

Scarlet Fever
DO THESE APPLY:

- A rash accompanies a sore throat
- You suspect scarlet fever

YES

CALL DOCTOR

NO

DIFFERENT SYMPTOMS?

see *Skin Symptoms*, p. 127

Fifth disease

A contagious childhood rash

When is a disease almost not a disease at all? When it's Fifth disease, the least noteworthy among the five most common contagious rashes of childhood.

Fifth disease has no symptoms except a rash, no complications, and needs no treatment. Its characteristic symptom is a "slapped cheek" appearance in children. This symptom is caused by a rash which is fine and pink, and usually begins on the cheeks and spreads to the backs of arms and legs. It gets brighter in response to heat. It can appear and disappear over the course of several weeks, but is usually gone in four or five days. For symptoms that may indicate other conditions, see *Skin Symptoms*, p. 127.

Fifth disease is highly contagious. The rash appears six to 14 days after exposure, but causes no problems. A child with the disease usually does not run a fever or feel sick. No self-care is needed. If a child develops a fever with a rash, it probably is not Fifth disease.

Adults with Fifth disease may develop joint pain and a mild pink color to their cheeks. Joint pain may last one to three months, and is usually reduced with an anti-inflammatory such as ibuprofen. Because it poses a slight risk to developing fetuses, pregnant women should avoid exposure if possible and see their doctor if exposure does occur.

3

OTHER COMMON CONCERNS

Croup

A bark usually worse than its bite

Croup is a viral infection of the respiratory tract characterized by a hoarse cough (seal-like "bark") that subsides during the day, and difficulty breathing — especially at night. In addition, there may be a low-grade fever, and hoarseness that may be preceded by a cold or mild upper-respiratory infection.

Because it usually occurs in children under 3 or 4 years of age, and often at night, croup can be an alarming experience for parents. Fortunately, croup can frequently be treated at home and symptoms generally improve within a week or so.

What you can do

OPEN AIR PASSAGES FOR EASIER BREATHING

- Expose the child to humidity. Bathroom steam is a good source of warm, moist air. Let the shower run with hot water, then bring the child into the bathroom with you. Shut the door and hold the child on your lap for several minutes in the steamy room.

- Moisten the air with a cool-mist vaporizer. Cool-mist vaporizers eliminate the danger of scalding associated with vaporizers that heat water for steam.

- Take your child into the cool night air.

If one of these approaches does not bring relief and the child is not worsening, try another approach.

MONITOR YOUR CHILD'S IMPROVEMENT

Croup is usually relieved with simple home remedies. A more serious, but less common illness with similar symptoms, called *epiglottitis,* does not respond to these self-care techniques. The child should receive medical attention immediately if epiglottitis is suspected. It is caused by a bacterial infection and generally affects children over 3 years old. Children with epiglottitis have extreme difficulty breathing. They drool and assume a characteristic position with their head tilted forward, chin jutted out, while gasping for air.

Repeated bouts of croup may be caused by an underlying bacterial infection or congenital malformation of the air passages. You can rest easier, however, knowing croup usually disappears by age 7, when the child's air passages have matured.

Final notes

Due to the alarming cough and the late hour croup often strikes, many parents panic when faced with the child's first case. Try to stay calm and begin the self-care steps suggested under *What You Can Do.*

see *Know What To Do,* p. 102

Croup

DO THESE APPLY:

- Stops breathing, turns blue

  see *CPR*, p. 20

- Barking cough, increased breathing difficulty
  AND high-pitched wheezing sound when
  breathing

- Muscles between ribs move inward when child
  inhales (*retractions*)

- Episodes of restlessness or "air hunger,"
  especially if followed by episodes of fatigue

- Child assumes characteristic position of
  epiglottitis with chin jutting out as they
  breathe through mouth, with drooling and
  difficulty breathing

- Markedly pale skin

- Possibility of foreign body obstructing airway

  see *Choking,* p. 24

YES

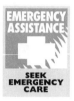

EMERGENCY ASSISTANCE

SEEK EMERGENCY CARE

--- **NO** ---

- No signs of improvement after 15 minutes
  of self-care

- Marked improvement with self-care, but
  problem continues for more than one hour

- Marked improvement with self-care and child
  is less than 3 months old

YES

CALL DOCTOR NOW

--- **NO** ---

see *What You Can Do*

APPLY SELF-CARE

Ear infections

A common childhood illness

Most children get a middle ear infection (*otitis media*) at least once, if not several times, by the time they are 3 years old. In addition, it is possible to get ear infections at any age (for adults, see *Middle Ear Infection*, p. 193).

Ear infections usually strike after an upper respiratory infection, when the tubes between the ear and the throat (*eustachian tubes*) swell and close. As a result, fluid and mucus gather in the middle ear and bacteria breed. Infants and young children are most susceptible to ear infections because their eustachian tubes are shorter and not fully developed.

Infants and young children who cannot talk may tug on the ear as a sign of ear pain. Other symptoms may include fever, decreased hearing, difficulty sleeping and fussiness.

Prevention

- Breast-feed your baby. This will pass on a natural immunity to infection.
- Feed infants in an upright or semi-upright position to prevent milk from getting into the eustachian tube. Don't allow babies to fall asleep with a bottle.
- Teach children to blow their nose gently, with their mouth open.
- Avoid exposing children to cigarette smoke. Irritation and inflammation caused by smoke can narrow the eustachian tubes and contribute to ear problems.

What you can do

- See your doctor for evaluation. Antibiotics are the standard treatment for middle ear infection (make sure the child takes all the prescribed medication).
- Acetaminophen (Tylenol) may help relieve discomfort. **NEVER give aspirin to children/teenagers. It can cause Reye's syndrome, a rare but often fatal condition.**
- Encourage the child to get as much rest as possible and drink plenty of clear fluids.

3

- Place a warm washcloth, warm water bottle or heating pad (set on low) directly on the affected ear. Do not leave a child alone with a heating pad.

- Use a cool-mist vaporizer to moisturize the air, which helps control levels of mucus.

- Do not insert **any** type of object into the ear to relieve itching or pain.

Final notes

If your child suffers from recurrent ear infections, you and your doctor may want to discuss the possibility of:

- Prophylactic antibiotics (a preventive, low-dose antibiotic taken daily throughout the season the child is most prone to ear infections); or

- Surgical insertion of tiny tubes (*tympanostomy tubes*) through the eardrum to improve drainage and ventilation of the middle ear

---

WORRIED ABOUT HEARING LOSS?

While children may suffer temporary and minor hearing loss during and immediately following an ear infection, there is seldom any permanent hearing loss if prompt medical treatment is provided.

Pressure caused by an ear infection can also cause an eardrum to rupture (see *Ruptured Eardrum,* p. 194). A single rupture is not serious, but repeated ruptures may cause hearing loss.

know
WHAT
TO DO

Ear infections

DO THESE APPLY:

- **Ear pain accompanied by headache, fever and stiff neck** (see *Meningitis*, p. 271)

YES ▶

EMERGENCY
ASSISTANCE

SEEK EMERGENCY CARE

─── **NO** ───

- **Infant less than 3 months old has fever of 101° F or greater**
- **White-to-yellow or foul-smelling ear discharge**

YES ▶

CALL DOCTOR NOW

─── **NO** ───

- **Ear infection is suspected**
- **Infant 3 - 6 months old has fever of 101° F or higher**
- **Ear pain lasts more than an hour**
- **Symptoms increase — or fail to improve — after two or three days of antibiotic treatment**
- **Stuffy ears or hearing loss persists, without other symptoms, more than 10 days after cold clears up**

YES ▶

Dr. Smith

CALL DOCTOR

─── **NO** ───

see *What You Can Do*

For adults, see *Earaches/Stuffiness*, p. 193; *Ear Discharge*, p. 197; *Fever*, p. 112

APPLY SELF-CARE

Object in the nose

Swelling and discharge are clues

Young children place nearly everything they touch in their mouths, but sometimes strange objects find their way into young noses, too.

Note the symptoms

- Foul-smelling yellow or gray-green nasal discharge, often from one nostril
- Swelling of nose
- Nasal tenderness

What you can do

- Pinch the opposite nostril and let the child try to blow the object out.
- If you can see the object, carefully use tweezers to remove it while holding the child's head still. Be sure you don't push the object further inside the nose.
- Use a spray nasal decongestant in the affected nostril to reduce swelling.
- Call the doctor if you're unable to retrieve the object.

Colic

A mysterious misery

Babies with colic seem to have an internal alarm — and when it goes off you can be assured of hours of seemingly endless crying. This nerve-fraying condition is quite common among infants; about 25% of newborns will become "colicky" between 2 and 6 weeks of age.

It's not clear what causes colic. Current evidence indicates gastrointestinal problems are not to blame for colic, and it's unlikely that milk allergies are the cause, either. If your child is allergic to milk, other symptoms will appear, such as vomiting, diarrhea or eczema (see index for these topics).

While lengthy periods of crying are the most prominent symptom of colic, excessive crying can signal other problems, too. If your baby cries frequently or for long periods and has a fever or diarrhea, something other than colic is responsible and your baby should be seen by a doctor.

Colicky babies may have gas or an enlarged stomach right after feeding. When they cry, they may pull their legs up to their stomachs or stiffen and extend them. Colicky babies are usually healthy and are considered to have colic only when all other causes for prolonged crying have been ruled out. Your pediatrician can help you decide if colic is the culprit.

What you can do

FOR YOUR BABY

- If you are breast-feeding, talk with your doctor about your intake of milk and milk products. Avoid spicy foods, sugar and alcohol.

- If bottle-feeding, make sure bottle nipples are large enough to drip one drop of formula per second.

- Burp the baby often. Crying often stops after the baby burps or passes gas.

- Be sure your baby is getting enough to eat. It takes about two hours for a baby to digest a feeding. If the crying occurs less than two hours after feeding, the baby is probably not really hungry. Try steps other than feeding to calm your infant.

- Use a pacifier to soothe the infant between feedings.

- Place the infant on its stomach over your knees or forearm to ease discomfort.

- Use motion, such as walking, rocking, strolling or swinging, to comfort your baby.

FOR YOU

- Find a reliable sitter and enjoy an evening away once a week.

- It's OK occasionally to let the baby cry while you try to relax. However, don't let a newborn cry alone for more than 15 minutes.

- Know that colic is not the result of something you have done — it simply happens.

Final notes

Colic seems to last forever, but take heart: most infants suddenly end their crying bouts when they reach 3 to 4 months of age.

Colic

DO THESE APPLY:

- Infant has diarrhea, vomiting or constantly distended stomach

  see *Diarrhea,* p. 258

- If fever, see *Fever,* p. 112

YES

CALL DOCTOR

NO

see *What You Can Do*

APPLY SELF-CARE

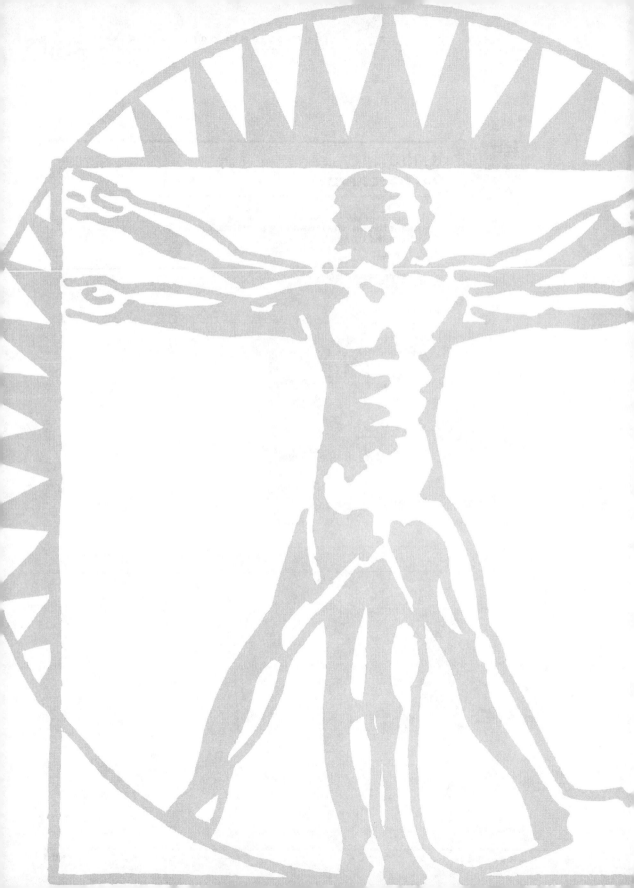

Chief concerns

4

NEUROLOGICAL

Fever

A symptom of fighting infection

Fever is a symptom — not an illness — that indicates the body is fighting an infection. It is an elevation in body temperature above "normal," which can vary in individuals from 96.8° F to 99.6° F.

Under healthy circumstances, your temperature varies throughout the day. It is lowest in the morning and highest in late afternoon. It is also normal for temperatures to rise due to hormonal changes during a woman's monthly menstrual cycle, anxiety, consumption of food and wearing heavy clothing.

Adults are considered to have a fever if their oral temperature is higher than 100° F. Children have a fever if their rectal temperature is higher than 100° F.

Note your symptoms

Generally, fever is caused by viruses, bacterial infections, fungi or parasites. Fever can also result from inflammatory diseases (like lupus and rheumatoid arthritis) and from cancers, such as Hodgkin's disease and kidney cancer.

Other physical signs of fever include:

• Feeling hot or cold

• Shivering

• Headache

• Muscle aches

• Joint pains

• General malaise

Since it is difficult for a young child to tell you that they have a fever, look for symptoms that may indicate fever:

- Uncharacteristic or high-pitched cry
- Child is inconsolable
- Difficulty rousing child
- Pale and/or bluish skin
- Symptoms of dehydration (see *Dehydration*, p. 262)
- Diminished activity
- Newborns may become lethargic, develop blotchy skin and alter their eating patterns

What you can do

Recent studies suggest that fever probably plays a role in combating infection. In other words, it's not always a bad thing. But it can be very uncomfortable, so most people prefer to minimize their discomfort with remedies such as acetaminophen (Tylenol), aspirin and ibuprofen.

- If medication is prescribed, follow your doctor's instructions and be sure to report any new symptoms.
- Good hygiene, particularly handwashing, is important in preventing infectious illnesses that cause fever.
- Warm (but never cold) baths or showers can also help to lower fever. Cool sponge baths may help in the case of a high fever — 102° F or higher. If fever is high, remove clothes and apply cool cloths to the head and chest. Sponging with lukewarm (not cold) water can also be effective. **Never give a child an alcohol bath.**
- Read all package instructions carefully to determine the proper dosage of medications for children. Dosage is based on both weight and age.
- Children with contagious illnesses should be kept home from school or day care.
- Immunization is an important step in preventing fever-related illnesses in children (see *Immunization Schedule*, p. 377).
- **NEVER give aspirin to children/teenagers. It can cause Reye's syndrome, a rare but often fatal condition.** Children and teenagers who take aspirin when they have chicken pox or flu are at a higher risk of developing Reye's syndrome. Since these illnesses, in the early

stages, can often be mistaken for some other ailment, it is recommended that parents always give children and teenagers acetaminophen (Tylenol) instead of aspirin to avoid this risk.

FEBRILE SEIZURES

A child with a high fever may experience a *febrile seizure* (also called a *convulsion*). Typically, the child suddenly loses consciousness, their arms and legs become rigid, and rhythmic twitching begins after a few seconds.

These seizures usually stop on their own in less than five minutes. They are associated with abnormal activity in the brain's nerve cells and tend to occur when the temperature is rapidly rising or falling. While frightening, they are relatively common and are not usually associated with long-term complications.

Cooling the child very quickly will NOT stop the seizure or prevent further seizures. NEVER leave an infant or child unattended in a bathtub, especially if there is a history of seizures.

If an infant has a seizure:

- Time the seizure. Do not move the baby or restrain movement.
- Breathing may stop momentarily; the baby should start breathing again independently in 30 to 60 seconds.
- Keep your fingers, pacifiers and other objects out of the mouth. Infants may bite their tongue, but will not swallow it.
- If vomiting occurs, place the baby on its stomach or side, never on its back.
- If breathing becomes labored, gently pull the jaw and chin forward by placing two fingers behind each corner of the jaw.
- After the seizure, **call your doctor**.

If a child older than 1 year has a seizure:

- Time the seizure. Lay the child down, removing any nearby objects that could cause injury. Do not restrain movement.
- Roll the child on its side to prevent the tongue from blocking the airway and to prevent choking.
- After the seizure, **call your doctor**.

Fever in adults

DO THESE APPLY:

- **Fever accompanies severe headache, stiff neck, lethargy or mental confusion**
- **Fever higher than 104° F that does not lower with self-care**
- **Fever accompanied by seizure**

YES ▶

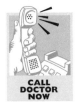

SEEK EMERGENCY CARE

──────────── **NO** ────────────

- **Fever and rapid breathing**

YES ▶

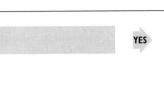

CALL DOCTOR NOW

──────────── **NO** ────────────

- **Fever shows no improvement in 72 hours**
- **Fever has lasted more than five days**
- **Low-grade fever persists for several weeks**

YES ▶

CALL DOCTOR

──────────── **NO** ────────────

see *What You Can Do*

see *Fever* in the index

APPLY SELF-CARE

For children, see *Know What To Do*, p. 116

Fever in children

DO THESE APPLY:

- **Fever accompanies severe headache, stiff neck, lethargy or mental confusion**
- **Fever in child less than 1 month old**
- **Fever higher than 101° F in child less than 3 months old**

YES →

SEEK EMERGENCY CARE

--- **NO** ---

- **Fever accompanied by seizure or rapid breathing**
- **Fever higher than 103° F**

YES →

CALL DOCTOR NOW

--- **NO** ---

- **Fever in child between 4 months and 1 year of age has lasted more than 24 hours**
- **Fever shows no improvement in 72 hours**
- **Fever has lasted more than five days**

YES →

CALL DOCTOR

--- **NO** ---

see *What You Can Do*

see *Fever* in the index

APPLY SELF-CARE

Tension headaches

Painful but common

Almost everyone gets tension headaches ranging from that dull ache to unbearable pain. They are caused by the stretching, or tension, of the outer lining of the brain, the skin and muscles that cover the skull, and the nerves that travel from the brain to the head and face. Tight muscles in the shoulders, back and neck can also cause tension headaches.

Tension headaches are frequently caused by emotional or physical stress. Figuring out the exact causes — or triggers — of your particular headaches can help you reduce or avoid them in the future. Situations that make you grit your teeth, tighten your shoulders or clench your fist may cause headaches. This list of causes is endless and could include commuting, loud noises, dealing with a difficult person, sitting in an uncomfortable desk chair, or getting too much or not enough sleep.

What you can do

- Aspirin, ibuprofen or acetaminophen (Tylenol) can blunt or eliminate pain. **NEVER give aspirin to children/teenagers. It can cause Reye's syndrome, a rare but often fatal condition.**

- Soak in a hot bath, or lie down in a darkened room with an ice bag on your forehead. For protection, place a washcloth between bare skin and ice.

- Get a massage.

- Take a nap.

- Exercise regularly and consider yoga, meditation or other muscle-relaxation techniques.

see *Know What To Do*, p. 121

4

Migraine headaches

Good news about managing pain

Migraine headaches can cause excruciating pain and prevent sufferers from carrying out daily activities. Migraines account for 2% to 7% of all headaches, affect more women than men and usually start to appear between the ages of 10 and 30. Some people experience fewer episodes as they grow older and may even enjoy a complete remission after age 50.

Migraines are believed to occur when blood vessels in the brain and scalp either close down, resulting in limited blood flow, or open way up, becoming swollen and taut.

The throbbing pain of a migraine is generally focused on one side of the head. Pain can bring a sensitivity to light, noise and movement. Other symptoms may include nausea, vomiting, diarrhea, frequent urination and blurred vision.

Factors that trigger migraines include glare from harsh light, stress, hunger, climatic changes, certain foods and beverages, oral contraceptives and medications that dilate (or open up) blood vessels, the menstrual cycle, physical or mental exhaustion, or too much or too little sleep.

If you are susceptible to migraines, you will generally experience several headaches a year (each lasting one to three days). If your headaches increase in severity or frequency, you may want to call your doctor. Medication may be prescribed to reduce your symptoms or help prevent chronic migraines. Sumatriptin is a relatively new drug that is proving helpful to many.

What you can do

The good news is that with the right combination of self-care techniques and appropriate medication, you can make a significant difference in your ability to manage, and possibly eliminate, this painful monster.

The key is to identify your triggers. Keeping a diary of your symptoms, possible triggers and which self-care techniques work and don't work provides helpful information for both you and your doctor.

You may be able to relieve or control pain from a migraine by:

- Lying down in a cool, dark, quiet room
- Putting an ice bag on your head. For protection, place a washcloth between bare skin and ice.
- Taking over-the-counter (OTC) painkillers such as aspirin, acetaminophen (Tylenol) or ibuprofen. (Any medication, food or beverage containing caffeine can cause a *rebound headache*.) **NEVER give aspirin to children/teenagers. It can cause Reye's syndrome, a rare but often fatal condition.**
- Practicing yoga, meditation or other muscle-relaxation techniques

see *Know What To Do*, p. 121

Cluster headaches

Similar to migraines

Cluster headaches are similar to migraines with a few differences. They occur mostly in men and are not necessarily inherited. They are one-sided like a migraine, but the throbbing, burning pain behind or above the eye becomes intense rapidly and lasts from 10 minutes to several hours. One to three attacks can occur in a 24-hour period, nausea and vomiting are rare, and nasal stuffiness may occur. They respond well to drugs that constrict the blood vessels such as *ergotamine*.

Headaches

DO THESE APPLY:

Headache is associated with:

- **Slurred speech**
- **Loss of coordination**
- **Double vision**
- **Numbness**
- **Rash, stiff neck or drowsiness**

  see *Meningitis*, p. 271

YES

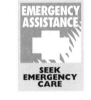

SEEK EMERGENCY CARE

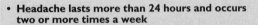 **NO**

- **Headache lasts more than 24 hours and occurs two or more times a week**
- **Headache is "worst ever"**
- **Pain really is "different" than other headaches**

Headache is associated with:

- **103° F fever but no other symptoms**
- **Nausea or vomiting, especially forceful vomiting**
- **Recent head injury**

  see *Head/Spinal Injury*, p. 60

YES

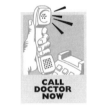

CALL DOCTOR NOW

NO

- **Child's headaches persist or occur several times a week**
- **Headache without obvious cause persists or doesn't improve with self-care**
- **Headaches increase in severity and frequency, and interfere with daily activities**
- **Pain relievers are needed several times a week**
- **Previously effective measures no longer provide same level of relief**
- **You suspect a migraine or cluster headache**

YES

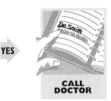

CALL DOCTOR

NO

see *What You Can Do, Tension Headaches*, p. 117

see *What You Can Do, Migraine Headaches*, p. 119

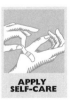

APPLY SELF-CARE

4

Dizziness/fainting

It can really floor you

Most of us have felt faint or dizzy at some time. There are many causes for these sensations — some minor and a few more serious. Most of these problems can be eased or eliminated with self-care.

Although many of these sensations seem similar, the differences in symptoms are important to help determine the cause and treatment. *Dizziness* is a sensation of spinning inside your head and can cause a loss of balance. *Fainting* (*syncope*) is the temporary decrease or loss of consciousness due to a momentary inadequate supply of blood to your brain. *Light-headedness* is a very mild faint or "woozy" feeling.

All of these sensations can be brought on by hunger, exhaustion, emotional upsets, severe pain, hot stuffy environments, laughing or urinating, drugs, alcohol, dehydration, variations in heart rhythm, a drop in blood pressure, standing up suddenly, or anything that momentarily decreases blood flow to your brain. *Vertigo* is when the room seems to move or spin around you, and is usually caused by a problem in the inner ear (see *Middle Ear Infection*, p. 193).

Prevention

- Eat well-balanced meals at regular intervals and snacks between meals if you are hungry.
- Work and exercise in moderate amounts. Stop and rest at intervals to avoid becoming exhausted.
- Drink eight glasses of water daily. Drink more in hot conditions.
- Limit your alcohol intake, especially in warm weather.
- Read about and learn the side effects of all medications and drugs you are taking.
- Get up slowly after sitting or lying in one position for a long time.
- Treat motion sickness with appropriate medications such as Dramamine or Bonine.
- Try to identify the cause of dizziness and avoid that activity in the future.

What you can do

DIZZINESS/FAINTING

- If you feel faint or dizzy, lie down and raise your legs above the level of your heart. If sitting, put your head down between your knees.
- Drink small amounts of liquid frequently if dehydrated (see *Dehydration,* p. 262).
- Move to a cool area if you're in a warm, stuffy environment.
- Check with your doctor about side effects of medication.

VERTIGO

- Lie quietly in a darkened room.
- Avoid sudden movements.
- Focus on one object or keep eyes closed to help ease spinning sensation.

see *Know What To Do,* p. 126

Weakness/fatigue

When you're just not up to par

Although they are often discussed together, weakness and fatigue are two distinctly different problems.

Weakness is a decrease in your physical ability or an increase in difficulty moving one or more muscles. It is usually the more serious symptom, especially when it involves a large group of muscles such as an arm or a leg, or one whole side of the body. Temporary or prolonged weakness in one part of the body may be a warning of injury to the nervous system or a stroke.

Fatigue is a feeling of weariness, exhaustion or decrease in energy. Causes may include stress, sudden change in physical activity level, change in medication, limited or altered sleep, exposure to toxic chemicals, recovery from a major health or emotional event, depression, poor nutrition or excessive alcohol intake. In many cases, symptoms can be treated and relieved through self-care within two months.

CHRONIC FATIGUE SYNDROME

If other conditions are ruled out, the diagnosis of Chronic Fatigue Syndrome (CFS) may be made. Formerly called "Epstein-Barr Virus Syndrome," CFS is a flu-like illness. In addition to prolonged and extreme fatigue, other symptoms include a sore throat, fever around 100° F, swollen lymph nodes, muscle aches and weakness, headache and emotional problems.

There are no definitive tests for CFS and no cure has been found. Treatment is focused on relieving the symptoms. Support is an important part of therapy, and many support groups are available.

Prevention

Prevention and self-care for problems related to weakness and fatigue include:

- Exercise regularly. Include exercises which strengthen and tone muscle and improve aerobic endurance (see *Staying Active*, p. 372).

- Eat a well-balanced diet that is high in fiber and low in fat (see *Eating Right*, p. 373).

- Improve your sleeping habits (see *Insomnia*, p. 353).
- Deal with any feelings of depression (see *Depression*, p. 355).
- Limit your intake of alcohol, caffeine and nicotine.
- Provide variety in your activities and interests.
- Avoid exhaustion by scheduling time for rest and relaxation.

What you can do

- Follow the prevention guidelines above.
- You can help your doctor diagnose the cause of your fatigue by keeping track of when the feeling started, when it occurs or is most intense, anything that seems to make it worse or better, if others in your home or work setting have similar problems, and any other changes or symptoms you notice.
- Listen to your body. Notice the effect drugs, activities and stress have on you.
- Be patient. It may take six to eight weeks of practicing prevention and self-care guidelines regularly before you feel strong and energetic again.

Final notes

Prolonged or extreme fatigue that does not respond to self-care may be a sign of a more serious problem. Chronic fatigue is a symptom often found in many diseases such as diabetes, hypothyroidism, anemia, mononucleosis, lupus, heart disease and rheumatoid arthritis, to name a few.

see *Know What To Do,* p. 126

Dizziness/fainting/weakness/fatigue

DO THESE APPLY:

- **Complete loss of consciousness**

  Lay victim down in safe place. Check for breathing and pulse. Start CPR if needed (see CPR, p. 20).

  see *Unconsciousness*, p. 40

- **Weakness or dizziness accompanied by headache, loss of hearing, blurred vision, weakness or numbness in arms or legs, sudden weakness on one side of the body**

  Have victim lie down or sit in supported position. Check breathing and keep airway clear.

- **Symptoms follow head injury**

  see *Head/Spinal Injury*, p. 60

YES

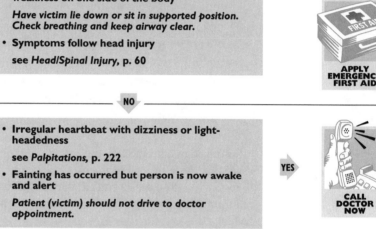

SEEK EMERGENCY CARE

APPLY EMERGENCY FIRST AID

NO

- **Irregular heartbeat with dizziness or light-headedness**

  see *Palpitations*, p. 222

- **Fainting has occurred but person is now awake and alert**

  Patient (victim) should not drive to doctor appointment.

YES

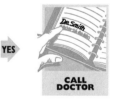

CALL DOCTOR NOW

NO

- **Dizziness not relieved with prevention or self-care**

- **Vertigo continues or recurs**

- **Dizziness may be caused by prescribed medication**

- **Weakness or fatigue do not improve after two to four weeks of self-care**

YES

CALL DOCTOR

NO
---

see *What You Can Do, Dizziness/Fainting*, p. 123

see *What You Can Do, Weakness/Fatigue*, p. 125

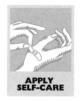

APPLY SELF-CARE

SKIN CONCERNS

SKIN SYMPTOMS

Rash	Appearance/ Location	Itching	Fever	Other Symptoms/ Comments
General Skin Conditions				
Acne p. 137	Red pimples, cysts, blackheads: on face, back, chest	No	No	Pimples may become whiteheads, may have general skin redness
Dandruff p. 133	White to yellow to red, some crusting: on scalp, eyebrows, groin	Occasional	No	Fine, oily scales and flaking
Eczema p. 130	Red; cracking and thickening of dry areas: on elbows, wrists, knees, cheeks	Moderate to intense	No	Moist, oozing, water-filled blisters
Impetigo p. 144	Shallow sores that have gold crusty surface color: on arms, legs (face first, then rest of body)	Occasional	Maybe	Weepy blisters form the crusty appearance
Psoriasis p. 131	Thick, silvery skin patches: often on knees, elbows, scalp	Moderate to intense	No	Symptoms come and go over weeks to months
Shingles p. 83	Small, fluid-filled blisters: usually on one side of body (most often the torso), accompanied by sharp nerve pain	Intense	Maybe	Blisters rupture, forming yellow, crusty scabs
Fungal Rashes				
Athlete's Foot p. 148	Colorless to red: between toes	Mild to intense	No	Cracks, scaling, oozing blisters
Jock Itch p. 147	Patches of redness, scaling and raised areas that ooze: on groin	Mild to intense	No	Penis and scrotum usually not involved
Ringworm p. 146	Red, slightly raised rings: located anywhere, including nails, scalp	Occasional	No	Fungus can cause hair loss and patchy bald spots

SKIN SYMPTOMS

Rash	Appearance/ Location	Itching	Fever	Other Symptoms/ Comments
Allergic Reactions				
Hives p. 139	Welt-like elevations, surrounded by redness: located anywhere	Intense	No	Reaction to an allergen; many possible causes
Poison Ivy/ Poison Oak	Red, elevated blisters: on any exposed area	Intense	No	Oozing; some swelling; rash begins 12 - 48 hrs. after contact with plant (also spread by pets, contaminated clothing, smoke from burning plants) and may persist for up to two weeks; to treat, clean affected skin area with soap and water, bathe with Aveeno powder
Rashes caused by chemicals p. 130	Red, possibly blisters: on any exposed area	Moderate to intense	No	Oozing and/or swelling
Childhood Rashes/Illnesses				
Baby Rashes p. 82	see *Baby Rashes* chart			
Chicken Pox p. 83	Red rash progresses from flat to raised, then blisters to crusts: may start anywhere, most prominent on torso and face	Intense during pustular stage	Yes	Mild, generalized ill feeling
Rubella (German Measles) p. 86	Light red; flat or slightly raised: first on face, then torso, then extremities	No	Yes	Swollen glands behind ears; occasional joint pain
Measles p. 89	Pink, then red, flat: first on face, then chest and abdomen, then arms and legs	None to mild	Yes	Preceded by fever, cough, red eyes

SKIN SYMPTOMS

Rash	Appearance/ Location	Itching	Fever	Other Symptoms/ Comments
Childhood Rashes/Illnesses				
Roseola p. 95	Pink and flat, with occasional bumps: first on torso, then arms and neck; slight on face and legs	No	Yes	High fever for three days, then rash appears
Scarlet Fever p. 97	Red, flat, like sandpaper: first on face, then elbows; spreads in 24 hours to entire body	No	Yes	Sore throat; skin peeling afterwards, especially on palms of hands
Fifth Disease p. 99	Red and flat, lacy appearance: first on face, then arms and legs, then rest of body	No	No	Slapped-cheek appearance, rash can come and go

Eczema and psoriasis

Itching for some relief?

Eczema, also known as *dermatitis*, is characterized by dry, scaly and itchy skin common to the face, neck, hands, elbows, wrists and/or knees. It is caused by the inability of the skin to retain enough water. Causes range from contact with detergents or other harsh substances (also called *contact dermatitis*) to emotional stress. Often, the cause of eczema is unknown.

A common form of eczema is called *atopic dermatitis*. You're a likely candidate if you have a personal or family history of asthma, hay fever or some other allergy. Recent studies suggest that certain foods — such as citrus fruits, wheat, eggs and nuts — might also be responsible for some cases of eczema.

Eczema is rare in infants under 2 months old, but if it does develop, it can be severe. Because infants can't scratch themselves with their fingers, they may rub itchy areas against their bed sheets, causing redness.

What you can do

- Avoid drying out the skin. Limit baths and showers and the use of soap. Use an unscented moisturizer.

- Use hypo-allergenic makeup, or none at all. Wear rubber gloves for dishwashing and other household chores. Wear cotton clothing (wool and synthetic materials may be irritating). Sweat aggravates eczema, so wear lightweight, loose-fitting clothes, especially during exercise.

- Swimming in fresh or chlorinated pool water can aggravate eczema, but salt water is not harmful.

- Most complications result from scratching or rubbing. Trim nails to minimize the effects of scratching.

- Do not apply anesthetic lotions or antihistamine creams unless your doctor prescribes them; they can actually increase irritation. For the worst areas, try using a cool gauze dressing soaked in diluted Burrow's solution, which is available in most drugstores. Apply the dressing three times a day for about 15 minutes.

PSORIASIS

Eczema can be confused with other skin conditions, such as *psoriasis,* another chronic skin condition. Psoriasis appears as silvery skin patches or *plaques* which are often on the knees, elbows and scalp. Normally, skin cells mature and are shed once a month. With psoriasis this occurs at a much faster rate, every three to four days. Because the *dermis* (lower layer of skin cells) is dividing so rapidly, dead cells accumulate in thicker-than-normal patches on the *epidermis* (skin's outermost layer). The symptoms of this chronic disease typically come and go over weeks or months and then disappear altogether.

As many as 4 to 5 million Americans cope with psoriasis. Although there is no cure, the right therapy can help control symptoms. Care is individualized and based on the severity of symptoms. Treatment may consist of self-care, *phototherapy* (exposure to ultraviolet or infrared light) and a variety of medications to help relieve the scaling.

What you can do

- Bathe daily to help soak off the scales.
- Avoid hot water or harsh soap. Anything that is drying to your skin will worsen psoriasis.
- Use an unscented moisturizer that does not contain lanolin.
- Treat small patches with occasional use of hydrocortisone cream.
- Try medicated shampoos (such as Head & Shoulders, Selsun blue and Capitrol) for scalp psoriasis.

If you think you have psoriasis, consult your doctor for a treatment plan that is best for your symptoms. If you've been diagnosed with psoriasis and your current treatment is no longer working, call your doctor. There are new products being developed which may help.

see *Know What To Do,* p. 132

Eczema and psoriasis

DO THESE APPLY:

- **Signs of infection:**
    - **Redness around the area or red streaks leading away**
    - **Swelling**
    - **Warmth or tenderness**
    - **Pus**
    - **Fever of 101° F or higher**
    - **Tender or swollen lymph nodes**

YES

**CALL
DOCTOR
NOW**

NO

- **Eczema sores become crusty or develop weepy discharge**
- **No improvement after one week of treatment or symptoms worsen**
- **Itching makes sleeping difficult despite self-care**
- **Eczema or psoriasis interferes with daily functions or causes increased emotional stress**

YES

**CALL
DOCTOR**

NO

see *What You Can Do*, pp. 130, 131

History of allergies? see *Allergies*, p. 210

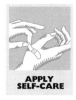

**APPLY
SELF-CARE**

DIFFERENT SYMPTOMS?

see *Skin Symptoms*, p. 127

Dandruff

It's a flaky, scaly scalp

Dandruff, or *seborrhea*, is a common condition characterized by flaky scaling of the scalp. Genetic factors play a role in determining who will suffer from dandruff, and climate can cause the onset of dandruff or more persistent symptoms (dandruff is more severe in winter when indoor air is dry). A yeast normally found in hair follicles may be responsible for many cases.

Symptoms similar to dandruff can be caused by psoriasis, poison ivy, poison oak, lice, eczema and ringworm (see index for these topics).

What you can do

- Use a dandruff shampoo (such as Head and Shoulders, Sebutone, Denorex, or one with salicylic acid) daily or every other day until symptoms improve.

- Once the dandruff improves, continue using dandruff shampoo twice a week to keep it under control.

- For severe scaling and redness, your doctor may prescribe medication containing fluocinolone acetonide or triamcinolone acetonide to be rubbed into the scalp twice a day.

- *Imidazoles*, or anti-yeast compounds, may be effective in treating severe dandruff in some cases.

see *Know What To Do*, p. 134

Dandruff

DO THESE APPLY:

- **You are immunocompromised with severe symptoms and/or dandruff is spreading to other areas of the body**
- **Symptoms become more severe, over-the-counter (OTC) medications fail to relieve**
- **Symptoms spread to face, along hairline, behind and in ears, on chest**

YES ▶

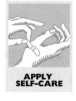

CALL DOCTOR

— **NO** —

- **Dry or greasy scaling of scalp**

see *What You Can Do*

YES ▶

APPLY SELF-CARE

Hair loss

Age and genetics are common causes

Hair is constantly being lost and replaced by your body. By far the most common reason for hair loss, or *alopecia*, is male-pattern baldness in which hair replacement fails to keep up with hair loss.

CAUSES

The cause of hair loss is often indicated by the way it falls out and the condition of the scalp. In *male-pattern baldness*, typically the hair loss starts with a receding hairline, continuing until only a horseshoe-shaped area of hair remains around the head. The scalp looks healthy. Both aging and genetics play a part in balding, with as many as 60% of men over age 50 affected. *Female-pattern baldness*, which is a general thinning of hair at the crown or hairline, is also genetic and influenced by hormonal changes during or after menopause.

Sudden loss of hair in patches is called *alopecia areata*. The hair generally grows back normally within several months.

Hair that falls out in large clumps and uncovers a normal-looking scalp may be due to a rare condition called *generalized alopecia*. It can be alarming to see clumps of hair in the shower drain or on a pillow. Causes usually involve physical or emotional stress such as surgery, trauma, pregnancy, high fever or burns. The hair usually falls out three to four months after the stressful event and will eventually grow back.

Chemotherapy can cause complete or partial hair loss on the body, with hair almost always growing back when treatment ends. Some common medications that can cause significant hair loss include heparin, oral contraceptives, amphetamines and beta blockers.

Hair loss that develops over weeks, months or even years can be due to autoimmune disease (such as *systemic lupus*), infectious diseases (such as *syphilis*) or endocrine disorders (such as *thyroid disease*).

Hair loss that is accompanied by an inflamed or scaly scalp may be caused by *psoriasis* or *dandruff* (see *Dandruff*, p. 133). The hair usually thins because of the intense scratching or applied treatment. If hair loss leaves bald spots with a gray-green scale, *ringworm* (a fungal infection) should be suspected (see *Ringworm*, p. 146).

Some people, especially children, may develop a nervous hair-pulling habit that can lead to hair loss.

What you can do

Male- and female-pattern baldness can't be prevented, but the drug *minoxidil* (Rogaine) has been used with mixed results. When rubbed on the scalp, this expensive cream has sometimes slowed hair loss and generated new hair growth, but many have been disappointed with the results.

Another alternative is hair transplantation, but successful cosmetic results are not always achieved and the procedure is painful, time-consuming and expensive.

Hair loss

DO THESE APPLY:

- **Bald areas have grayish-green scale**
  see *Ringworm*, p. 146
- **Sudden or dramatic hair loss**
- **New hair fails to grow normally**
- **Bald spots are patchy, don't follow the normal progression of male/female-pattern baldness**
- **Hair loss causes persistent or severe anxiety or depression**
- **Skin does not appear normal in area of hair loss**
- **Habitual hair-pulling, especially in children**

YES

CALL DOCTOR

NO

see *What You Can Do*

APPLY SELF-CARE

Acne

Just about everyone gets it at one time or another

Acne vulgaris refers to a spectrum of skin eruptions — blackheads, whiteheads, pimples, cysts and nodules — that can be sore, painful or itchy. Few people escape adolescence without a pimple or two.

Acne begins when a fatty oil, called *sebum*, and dead cells are manufactured too quickly and clog the pores around small hair follicles. The results can range from whiteheads to blackheads and pimples.

Acne tends to occur in areas where there are high concentrations of these *sebaceous glands* — the face, neck, shoulders, and upper and center back. In both sexes, elevated secretion of androgen hormones during puberty stimulates these glands to produce extra sebum, increasing the likelihood of acne.

What you can do

PRACTICE SMART PERSONAL HYGIENE

- Use a cleansing agent or soap that dries the skin enough to cause minor shedding (avoid too much drying since this can cause further irritation).

- Use a clean washcloth — gently.

- Never scrub the skin. If acne is not too severe (skin is not infected, pussy or raw), cleansing with a gentle abrasive such as Buff-Puff may help.

- Always rinse thoroughly.

- Give yourself an occasional mini-steam bath by placing a warm, wet towel on your skin for 10 to 15 minutes. This will help open pores and allow deeper cleaning.

- For infants with acne, wash the face daily with a clean cloth, water and mild soap.

SKIN MEDICATIONS

Acne medications unblock pores by drying up oil and promoting peeling. Many are available without a prescription and come in solutions that help cover up redness and scarring. Sunlight may temporarily clear up skin, but it can have other damaging effects — especially if drying agents or antibiotics are being used.

A doctor can prescribe stronger versions of topical skin medications or a special formulation of vitamin A, called *retinoic acid* (Retin-A), and antibiotics. Vitamin A also may be prescribed for severe cases and should be taken only as directed by your doctor — too much of it can be toxic.

Final notes

Carefully follow the directions, warnings and precautions on any drugs you use. Call your doctor if you have questions. And be patient — it may take two to six weeks or more to see progress with any of these self-care treatments or medications.

know WHAT TO DO

Acne

DO THESE APPLY:

- • Large, painful acne cysts
- • Acne that is extremely irritating or embarrassing
- • Post-adolescent women who develop severe acne and facial hair
- • No signs of improvement after four to six weeks of self-care
- • Symptoms worsen despite self-care

YES ➜

CALL DOCTOR

— **NO** —

see *What You Can Do*

APPLY SELF-CARE

Hives

Itching to get your attention

Hives are an allergic reaction. They are red, itchy, raised welts on the skin that may vary in size from less than a quarter-inch to more than an inch. Hives appear after you have been exposed to something that causes your body's antibodies to react, prompting the release of *histamine* into the skin. Hives may appear immediately or a few days after exposure and may last a few minutes, several days or come and go at intervals for weeks.

Common causes of hives include foods such as eggs, milk, wheat, berries, pork, chocolate, shellfish, nuts and cheese (see *Food Allergies*, p. 210). Other triggers include molds, pollens, animal dander, insect bites, chronic infection, drugs, vaccines, heat, sunshine, cold, perfumes or stress.

You can react on the first exposure or after many contacts with the cause of your hives. It is often difficult to determine the cause, and mild cases are treated only to relieve symptoms. Allergy tests are done if the symptoms become severe and interfere with your normal activities or if your hives are accompanied by other signs of an allergic response.

Prevention

- Avoid foods, medications or contacts that may have caused hives in the past.
- Use insect repellent and extra caution when you are in areas that have insects you may be allergic to.
- Inform all your doctors and dentists of your allergies.
- Learn stress-management techniques if stress appears to be a trigger for your hives (see *Stress*, p. 349).

What you can do

- Relieve itching skin areas by applying cool, wet compresses soaked in ice water or Burrow's solution (available in most drugstores).
- Bathing in lukewarm water containing one-half to one cup of Aveeno powder, one cup of baking soda or finely ground oatmeal may ease itching in large areas.
- Try over-the-counter (OTC) oral antihistamines such as Benadryl or Chlor-Trimeton. Read the precautions on the label regarding drowsiness.
- Apply a very thin layer of over-the-counter (OTC) hydrocortisone cream on small areas. Do not use near your eyes, mouth or genitals.
- Cut nails short or wear cotton gloves at night to prevent harmful effects of scratching.
- Avoid the cause of your hives.

Hives

DO THESE APPLY:

Hives with:

- **Shortness of breath or difficulty breathing**
- **Wheezing**
- **Tightness in chest**
- **Dizziness**
- **Swelling or puffiness around eyes, mouth or throat**
- **Nausea**

see *Allergies*, p. 210

see *Wheezing*, p. 232

YES → **EMERGENCY ASSISTANCE** — **SEEK EMERGENCY CARE**

—— NO ——

- **Hives after a bee sting**
- **Large hives over most of the body**
- **Hives soon after starting new prescription drug; do not take another dose**

Watch for any other symptoms listed above.

YES → **CALL DOCTOR NOW**

—— NO ——

- **Hives with a fever of 100° F or higher**
- **Severe itching not relieved with self-care**
- **Hives continue or persist after two weeks of self-care**

  see *Prevention*

  see *What You Can Do*

YES → **CALL DOCTOR**

—— NO ——

- **Red, itchy, raised welts on skin**

  see *What You Can Do*

YES → **APPLY SELF-CARE**

DIFFERENT SYMPTOMS?

see *Skin Symptoms*, p. 127

4

Boils

Pain that gets your attention

A boil is a red, swollen, painful bump that looks like a large pimple. It is usually caused by an infected hair follicle in an area of your body that is under pressure or chafed.

Common sites for boils are the buttocks, groin, waistline, armpits, neck and face. Bacteria, most often *staphylococcus,* get blocked in the follicle and develop an abscess. The tissue around the follicle becomes tender and inflamed as it tries to wall off the infection. This forces the abscess outward until it ruptures on the skin surface and drains. If the wound is left open and clean, it can heal; if it closes off too soon, the pus pocket can form again.

Prevention

- For areas that are prone to boils, wash well with antibacterial soap. Dry thoroughly.

- Avoid clothing that is too tight. Eliminate chafing and ease pressure against your skin whenever possible.

- Keep clothes and personal linen of someone with a boil separate from the rest of the household to prevent spreading the infection.

What you can do

- Bathe with antibacterial soap to prevent boils from spreading.

- Apply warm, moist compresses to the boil for 20 to 30 minutes, four times a day. The moist heat will help bring the boil to a head and soften the skin to ease the rupture. This may take up to a week of compress treatments.

- ***Do not squeeze, scratch, cut or force the boil to drain.*** Any pressure or forced opening can push the bacteria deeper into the skin and spread the infection.

- Once the boil begins to drain, keep the wound open and clean, and:

  - Continue applying compresses at least three times a day.

  - Wash the area thoroughly with soap and water two times a day or as needed.

  - Apply antibacterial ointment and a sterile bandage after each compress treatment or whenever the old dressing becomes moist.

- Take aspirin or ibuprofen to ease pain and inflammation (follow the directions on the package). **NEVER give aspirin to children/ teenagers. It can cause Reye's syndrome, a rare but often fatal condition.**

- Watch for signs of infection:
  - Redness around the boil or red streaks leading away; swelling; warmth or tenderness; pus; fever of 101° F or higher; tender or swollen lymph nodes

Boils

DO THESE APPLY:

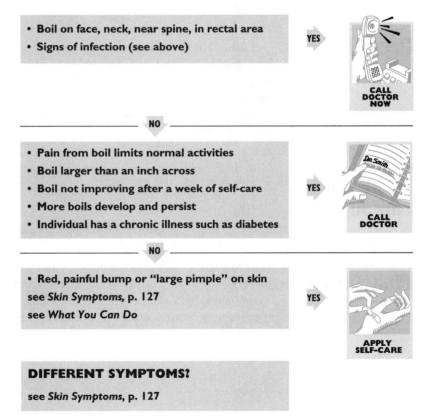

- **Boil on face, neck, near spine, in rectal area**
- **Signs of infection (see above)**

YES → CALL DOCTOR NOW

NO

- **Pain from boil limits normal activities**
- **Boil larger than an inch across**
- **Boil not improving after a week of self-care**
- **More boils develop and persist**
- **Individual has a chronic illness such as diabetes**

YES → CALL DOCTOR

NO

- **Red, painful bump or "large pimple" on skin**
  see *Skin Symptoms*, p. 127
  see *What You Can Do*

YES → APPLY SELF-CARE

DIFFERENT SYMPTOMS?

see *Skin Symptoms*, p. 127

Impetigo

A contagious skin infection

Impetigo is a highly contagious bacterial infection that frequently occurs around the mouth and nose, and is most common among children. It is characterized by itchy red sores on the face, legs or arms. The sores are first red and blistering, then ooze for several days forming a sticky, honey-colored crust. *Ecthyma* is a form of impetigo that causes deeper sores.

Impetigo often follows fungal infections, scabies, lice or other conditions that cause dermatitis. Sometimes insect bites cause impetigo (see index for these topics).

Most often, appropriate treatment leads to complete and rapid healing.

Prevention

The fluid inside the blisters contains the bacteria responsible for the condition. That means ruptured blisters can spread the infection. Excessive scratching can also spread the infection to other parts of the body or to other people. Do not share towels, clothing or razors with anyone until the infection is completely gone. Keep fingernails short to minimize scratching. Minimize personal contact with others until the infection clears.

What you can do

- Soak off crusts with warm water and washcloth.
- Wash the affected area gently several times a day with antibacterial soap or cleanser.
- Use an over-the-counter (OTC) topical antibiotic ointment.

Final notes

The most serious side effect of impetigo is a rare kidney condition called *glomerulonephritis.* It causes urine to turn dark brown and is often accompanied by headaches and elevated blood pressure. If you have these symptoms, see your doctor. Most people make a complete recovery.

Impetigo
DO THESE APPLY:

- Impetigo is worsening or not responding to treatment and you develop symptoms of a systemic infection (fever, malaise, fatigue, nausea)
- An infant under 6 months of age has symptoms
- Signs of infection develop after two to three days of self-care: redness around the area or red streaks leading away, swelling, warmth or tenderness, pus, fever of 101° F or higher, tender or swollen lymph nodes

YES →

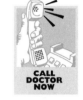

CALL DOCTOR NOW

NO

- Sores do not begin to heal after 24 to 48 hours of self-care
- Impetigo doesn't begin to heal or worsens after two to three days of oral antibiotic treatment
- Nostril, lip, face areas swell and become tender
- Impetigo covers two inches in diameter or more
- Anyone in your family or neighborhood has had glomerulonephritis recently
- An infant over 6 months of age or young child appears to have impetigo

YES →

CALL DOCTOR

NO

see *What You Can Do*

APPLY SELF-CARE

DIFFERENT SYMPTOMS?

see *Skin Symptoms*, p. 127

Ringworm

It's not really a worm

Oddly enough, ringworm has nothing to do with worms. It is a fungal infection of the nails, skin or scalp, caused by the same group of fungi that is responsible for athlete's foot (see *Athlete's Foot*, p. 148) and jock itch (see *Jock Itch*, p. 147). It gets its name from its characteristic red rings.

The infection can be spread from one person to another, from an animal to a person, or acquired by contact with contaminated soil, shoes, shower stalls and carpeting.

Ringworm typically begins as a small, pink, round patch which eventually turns red and grows into a ring shape. The center clears as the ring enlarges. Within a week or two, more patches may appear.

Prevention

Have all pets checked for ringworm before bringing them into your home, and teach children not to touch stray dogs or cats. Launder secondhand clothing. Always use your own towels and wear sandals in public showers, pools or locker rooms.

What you can do

Over-the-counter (OTC) medications applied to the skin are effective treatments for ringworm. Popular brands include Tinactin, Micatin and Lotrimin. Selsun Blue shampoo applied as a cream is an economical choice. Use small amounts two to three times a day, following directions on the container. Continue treatment for one week or more.

Ringworm thrives in warmth and moisture, so keep the infected area clean and dry. Wear loose, cotton clothing and clean all clothes in hot water and detergent. Avoid damp public areas, such as locker rooms and swimming pools.

see *Know What To Do*, p. 149

Jock itch

Once is enough

Jock itch affects boys and men. Symptoms include minor to intense itching in the groin area and, in more serious cases, patches of redness, scaling and raised areas that ooze. The penis and scrotum are usually not involved.

What you can do

Since this fungus thrives in warmth and moisture, your goal is to eliminate both. That means changing sweaty or soiled clothes as soon as possible, and washing underwear, jock straps and exercise clothes in hot water and detergent. Loose, cotton boxer shorts are better than tight shorts or briefs. Use a powder, such as cornstarch, two to three times a day to dust the groin area, especially after showering.

Nonprescription medications can be used, such as *tolnaftate* (Tinactin), *miconazole* (Micatin), or *clotrimazole* (Clotrimin). Be sure to follow directions on the container. You may need to continue use after symptoms are gone to prevent recurrence.

see *Know What To Do*, p. 149

4

Athlete's foot

Calls for persistent self-care

Athlete's foot, which can cause your feet to be red, itchy and irritated, is really ringworm that affects one in five Americans. These fungi typically spread from person to person in public areas such as showers and swimming pools.

Once it infects the feet, athlete's foot thrives in the warmth and moisture of shoes and socks. Other symptoms may include tenderness, soreness, scaling and a burning sensation. In severe cases, the skin between the toes or even the soles of the feet may become unnaturally soft, peel and even crack.

Prevention

Go barefoot when possible, or wear sandals or canvas shoes. Wear cotton socks to absorb moisture and change them every day. Alternate pairs of shoes so that they dry between wearings. Wear thongs in public locker rooms and showers.

What you can do

Keep your feet clean and dry. Wash them twice a day with soap and water, drying them completely, especially between the toes. After drying, sprinkle an over-the-counter (OTC) antifungal powder on them, such as Desenex and Zeasorb-AF.

If athlete's foot persists, try a nonprescription antifungal medication such as Miconazole cream (2%), Clotrimazole cream or lotion (1%), or Whitefield's tincture (especially effective for feet that are scaly or wet).

see *Know What To Do*, p. 149

Ringworm/jock itch/athlete's foot
DO THESE APPLY:

- For any signs of infection:
  - Redness around the area or red streaks leading away
  - Swelling
  - Warmth or tenderness
  - Pus
  - Fever of 101° F or higher
  - Tender or swollen lymph nodes

YES
CALL DOCTOR NOW

NO

- Symptoms of athlete's foot or other foot problems and are diabetic and/or have peripheral vascular disease
- Thickened, distorted, yellowish, crumbly toenails *(possible fungal infection of nails)*
- Symptoms of ringworm on scalp or on large areas of chest or abdomen
- Jock itch seems to spread to anal area
- Symptoms of any fungal problems persist or worsen after self-care
- Ringworm is not completely gone after four weeks of treatment

YES
CALL DOCTOR

NO

- Rash begins as small, round, pink patches
- Patches turn red and grow into ring shape
- Center of ring clears as it enlarges
see *What You Can Do, Ringworm,* p. 146
- Minor to intense groin itching
  see *What You Can Do, Jock Itch,* p. 147
- Red, itchy, irritated feet
  see *What You Can Do, Athlete's Foot,* p. 148

YES
APPLY SELF-CARE

Warts

They're usually harmless

Warts are small lumps that appear on the skin caused by a virus. They are very common, especially among young people. Warts are usually harmless and often disappear by themselves or with minimal treatment. But in some cases, warts may persist for years and in very rare instances, a wart may become cancerous.

Appearance and size of warts depend on their location and whether they are subjected to pressure, irritation or trauma. *Plantar warts* (flattened growths on the soles of the feet), for example, can be very painful because of the pressure of standing on them.

What you can do

Repeated applications of topical over-the-counter (OTC) medications will clear up many types of warts. For painful plantar warts, applying a donut-shaped pad to the area may provide temporary relief. Persistent plantar warts may require acid treatment or surgical removal by your doctor. Most warts disappear spontaneously within two years.

Final notes

For warts that do not respond to treatment with over-the-counter (OTC) medications, your doctor may remove them using various methods (which may cause scarring):

- Freezing with liquid nitrogen
- Acid treatment
- Electrical burning
- Laser surgery

know
WHAT TO DO

Warts
DO THESE APPLY:

- **Warts look infected after being irritated or knocked off**
- **You have warts in the anal or genital area**
  see *STD Chart*, p. 339
- **You have an abnormal growth on your skin and don't know what it is**
- **Warts on the face**
- **Painful warts**
- **Multiple warts**
- **Warts continue to be a concern and do not respond to self-care**

YES ▶

CALL DOCTOR

▼ **NO**

see *What You Can Do*

APPLY SELF-CARE

4

Scabies

Can spread easily through household

Scabies is a highly contagious condition caused by tiny parasitic creatures called *mites*. It is usually transmitted through skin-to-skin contact and spreads easily through households and schools.

The mites burrow into the skin and lay eggs just below its surface. The skin reacts with a rash and intense itching which is usually worse at night. Red track marks may be noted. These symptoms are commonly seen between the fingers, on the inside of wrists, armpits, genitalia and breasts.

Scratching may transmit bacteria already present on the skin into the open sores, resulting in a secondary bacterial infection.

What you can do

Elimite Cream (5% permethrin) is the recommended treatment for scabies. Follow the package instructions. Crotamiton (Crotan) also is effective but is not approved for use by children or pregnant women.

Medication should be applied all over the body except around the eyes, mouth, nose and vaginal or urethral opening. Itching may be relieved by cool baths, cortisone cream or ointment, calamine lotion, over-the-counter (OTC) pain relievers such as aspirin, ibuprofen or acetaminophen (Tylenol). **NEVER give aspirin to children/teenagers. It can cause Reye's syndrome, a rare but often fatal condition**. Itching may persist for one or two weeks after treatment.

know
WHAT
TO DO

Scabies

DO THESE APPLY:

- **Signs of infection:**
  - **Redness around the area or red streaks leading away**
  - **Swelling**
  - **Warmth or tenderness**
  - **Pus**
  - **Fever of 101° F or higher**
  - **Tender or swollen lymph nodes**

YES ▶

CALL DOCTOR NOW

NO

- **You think you may have scabies**
- **No improvement 72 hours after treatment**

YES ▶

CALL DOCTOR

NO

see *What You Can Do*

APPLY SELF-CARE

DIFFERENT SYMPTOMS?

see *Skin Symptoms*, p. 127

4

Lice

Scratch marks, swollen glands are signs

Pediculosis is a highly communicable infestation of small, white, blood-sucking insects called lice. The eggs are called *nits* and they usually attach themselves to hair close to the scalp or body. Pediculosis may result in swollen glands in the back of the neck and scratch marks behind the ears, along the hairline and on the neck. Hair may be matted and foul-smelling. Lice usually can't be seen without a magnifying glass.

Pediculosis is spread through direct personal contact or through sharing clothing or personal items with someone who is infested.

Lice are most common on the head or genital area but are also sometimes found on body hair, eyebrows, eyelashes and clothing. They can be common in overcrowded living conditions where there are inadequate facilities for good personal hygiene and clothes washing.

Head lice in school children are unrelated to hygiene or economic status, and are commonly found in schools, camps and other places where children share common space.

Genital lice (*crabs*) are frequently transmitted through sexual contact, but may also be acquired from infested toilet seats, towels, bedding or clothes.

Lice bites usually leave a tiny red spot, but scratching can cause larger sores to develop.

What you can do

- 1% *permethrin* (Nix Creme Rinse), available over-the-counter (OTC), is recommended for head lice. A single application is usually all that's needed.

- A-200 (pyrethrin), RID, Cuprex, all available over-the-counter (OTC), and Lindane, available by prescription, are remedies for lice. Lindane is not recommended for use on children under 2 or pregnant women, because it is potentially damaging to developing nerve tissue.

- *Malathion lotion* (Ovide) also can be used to treat head lice. Dry hair naturally after using because it is flammable.

- Lice in the eyelashes are treated with a thick layer of petroleum jelly, twice daily for eight days. If any nits are left, they can be removed with tweezers.

- Treat all exposed people at the same time to avoid reinfestations. Wash all possible sources of contamination such as brushes, clothing and bedding. Vacuum carpets and upholstered furniture.

see *Know What To Do,* p. 157

Bedbugs

They may be hiding in your bed

As you may have guessed, bedbugs spend most of their time in bed, hiding in the darkness of your sheets and blankets. Though related to lice, bedbugs are entirely different creatures. They are about one-quarter inch long and are wingless, red, oval bugs. They feed for 10 to 15 minutes a day, hate light and have a strong sense of when a warm body is approaching. They are very difficult to catch.

A bedbug bite is a firm lump or cluster, or firm lumps, found anywhere on the skin.

What you can do

To "sleep tight and not let the bedbugs bite," treat the bed and room where the bedbugs are located (they do not hide on the body or in clothing). Wash your bedding in hot water and follow the advice of your local health department.

see *Know What To Do*, p. 157

Lice/bedbugs

DO THESE APPLY:

- If you have lice and develop signs of infection:
    - Redness around the area or red streaks leading away
    - Swelling
    - Warmth or tenderness
    - Pus
    - Fever of 101° F or higher
    - Tender or swollen lymph nodes

YES → **CALL DOCTOR NOW**

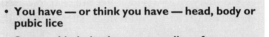
NO

- You have — or think you have — head, body or pubic lice
- Severe skin irritation or more lice after treatment
- Pregnant, lactating, or you suspect a child under 2 years old has lice

YES → **CALL DOCTOR**

NO

- Symptoms of bedbugs

  see *What You Can Do*, pp. 155, 156

YES → **APPLY SELF-CARE**

DIFFERENT SYMPTOMS?

see *Skin Symptoms*, p. 127

4

Tick bites

They need immediate attention

Ticks are small parasites related to spiders that embed themselves in the skin of humans and other animals, including household pets. Although tick bites are rarely harmful, ticks may transmit serious diseases such as *Rocky Mountain spotted fever* and *Lyme disease.*

Ticks are common in all outdoor areas of the United States and may be passed to people by their pets. Ticks frequently lodge in the scalp, nape of the neck, ankles, genital area or skin folds. They should be removed promptly and completely from people and household pets.

Tick bites often go unnoticed. Although small, ticks embedded in the skin are usually visible. Tick bites are characterized by itching; a small, hard lump on the skin; and redness surrounding the bite.

Prevention

- Avoid tick-infested areas, such as thickly wooded brush, whenever possible.

- Use an insect repellent on your skin whenever you plan to be outdoors for any length of time, especially in the warm months of spring and summer.

- Wear light-colored clothing.

- Wear long-sleeved shirts and long pants. Make sure your shirt is tucked inside your pants, and tuck your pants inside your boots or socks.

- After being in a known tick-infested area, check your body thoroughly and remove any ticks you find.

What you can do

NEVER SCRATCH A TICK BITE

The body of the tick may break off, leaving the head embedded in the skin.

What you can do

REMOVAL OF TICKS

Ticks should be removed carefully and promptly to help prevent the diseases they carry.

- With small tweezers, grip the tick as close to the surface of the skin as possible. Pull straight up and out using gentle, steady pressure. Do not squeeze the body of a tick, since this can increase the chance of getting a disease carried by ticks.

- Extract the tick slowly and firmly to assure complete removal.

- Clean the area of the tick bite with soap and water, then apply antiseptic.

Final notes

Lyme disease is usually transmitted by small deer ticks, common in summer and early fall. Symptoms develop three to 32 days after a bite. Common regions for this disease are the Atlantic Coast, Wisconsin, Minnesota, California and Oregon. However, sporadic cases have been reported in 46 states.

Rocky Mountain spotted fever is usually transmitted by wood ticks in the West and by dog ticks and lone star ticks in the East and Southeast. This disease generally occurs in warm weather and symptoms begin suddenly, two to 14 days after the bite.

see *Know What To Do,* p. 160

4

Tick bites
DO THESE APPLY:

- **You are unable to remove a tick or think part of the tick is still embedded**
- **Signs of infection:**
    - **Redness around the area or red streaks extending from the bite**
    - **Swelling**
    - **Warmth or tenderness**
    - **Pus**
    - **Fever of 101° F or higher**
    - **Tender or swollen lymph nodes**

YES → **CALL DOCTOR NOW**

───────────── **NO** ─────────────

- **Fever (103° F or higher), chills, malaise and fatigue, headaches, muscle aches, joint pain or rash up to three weeks after a tick bite**

  Lyme disease typically begins with a ringed rash that looks like a "bull's-eye."

- **Specific symptoms of tick-borne infection (see above), particularly if you or your pet spend time outside**

YES → **CALL DOCTOR**

───────────── **NO** ─────────────

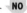

see *What You Can Do*

see *Insect Bites/Stings*, p. 55

APPLY SELF-CARE

Sunburn

A red-hot experience

A sunburn is a true burn of the outer layer of your skin. It is usually a *first-degree* burn causing skin redness and moderate discomfort. Severe sunburns with blisters, pain and swelling are *second-degree* burns and involve the deeper skin layer. Repeated sunburning and tanning have been shown to speed the skin's aging process and increase the risk of some cancers (see *Burns*, p. 30 and *Skin Cancer*, p. 163).

Prevention

- Use sunscreen with a sun protection factor (SPF) of at least 15. Apply sunscreen 15 minutes before exposure and reapply every two hours. If you are allergic to PABA, the active ingredient in many sunscreens, use non-PABA alternatives. Ask your pharmacist for recommendations.

- Check with your doctor or pharmacist to find out if any of your medications increase your skin's sensitivity to sunlight. If they do, use *extra* caution in the sun.

- Wear long sleeves and a hat with a broad brim or visor while you are in the sun.

- Drink extra fluids on sunny days, even if the temperature is not hot.

- Avoid the sun between 11 a.m. and 1 p.m. when the sun's rays are the strongest. Cloudy conditions do not screen out the rays that can burn your skin.

- Take sunburn precautions at high altitudes, in tropical climates, and around snow or water.

What you can do

- Cool compresses or baths may ease the discomfort. Adding one cup of baking soda or finely ground oatmeal to the bath water may increase the soothing effects.

- Take aspirin or ibuprofen to ease the pain and decrease inflammation. **NEVER give aspirin to children/teenagers. It can cause Reye's syndrome, a rare but often fatal condition.**

- Aloe vera gel or lotion may make your skin more comfortable.

- Avoid oil-based products, such as petroleum jelly, for the first 24 hours. They may actually retain the heat.
- Avoid products that contain anesthetic "caines" such as benzocaine. They may cause an allergic reaction in sensitive skin.
- Drink extra water and watch for signs of dehydration (see *Dehydration*, p. 262).
- Get extra rest and avoid exertion for 24 hours.

Sunburn
DO THESE APPLY:

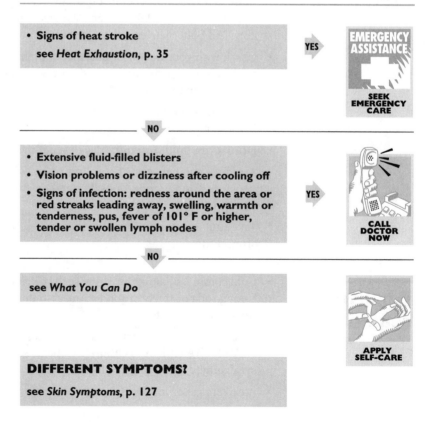

- **Signs of heat stroke**
  see *Heat Exhaustion*, p. 35

YES → SEEK EMERGENCY CARE

NO

- **Extensive fluid-filled blisters**
- **Vision problems or dizziness after cooling off**
- **Signs of infection: redness around the area or red streaks leading away, swelling, warmth or tenderness, pus, fever of 101° F or higher, tender or swollen lymph nodes**

YES → CALL DOCTOR NOW

NO

see *What You Can Do*

APPLY SELF-CARE

DIFFERENT SYMPTOMS?

see *Skin Symptoms*, p. 127

Skin cancer

Prevention, early detection are key

There are many types of skin cancer, but the three most common are:

Basal cell carcinoma: the most common type. It is a slow-growing cancer that forms in the outermost layer of the skin. If treated early, it is usually completely curable. If untreated, it can ultimately spread (*metastasize*) to bone and cartilage.

Squamous cell carcinoma: the second most frequent type. Out of 2,500 deaths annually from nonmelanoma skin cancer, 75% are from squamous cell carcinoma.

Malignant melanoma: the third most common and most deadly type of skin cancer. This is cancer of the *melanocyte*, the pigment cell of the skin. Unlike most other types of skin cancer, malignant melanoma can spread through the lymph system and the bloodstream. That's why it is very important that it be detected in the earliest possible stage. Over 70% of cases of early melanoma can be cured. However, the prognosis is not as favorable for cases that are treated in later stages. Other factors that influence the outcome of treatment include age and general health.

SOME CAUSES

The primary known cause of all types of skin cancer is exposure to ultraviolet (UV) radiation contained in sunlight. People who live in sunny climates and those with fair skin, freckles, blond or red hair, or blue eyes are at greatest risk. However, people with dark skin also can develop skin cancer. Some people with many moles (*nevi*) that contain abnormal (*dysplastic*) cells have an increased risk of developing melanoma.

Other factors that increase the risk of skin cancer include exposure to artificial sources of UV radiation (such as commercial tanning devices and phototherapy for certain skin disorders), concurrent use of certain drugs or cosmetics, immunosuppressive treatment, AIDS, hereditary disorders, and exposure to x-rays, uranium and a variety of chemicals.

Note your symptoms

Skin cancer forms without causing any symptoms of illness. Therefore, it's extremely important to be aware of the signs, especially in people with known risk factors.

Check your skin once a month for any skin irregularities. If you have any suspicious growths on your skin, have them checked by your doctor. A skin *biopsy*, in which part or all of the tissue from a mole or suspicious growth is removed for analysis, may be required. Biopsy is the only definitive test for melanoma.

MELANOMA

The "hallmark" sign of melanoma is a change in the size or shape of a mole. "ABCD" is an abbreviation used to make it easy to remember the four basic signs of possible melanoma:

- **A**symmetry — The shape of one half of a mole doesn't match the other.
- **B**order — The edges are ragged, notched or blurred.
- **C**olor — The color is uneven and shades of black, brown or tan are present. Areas of white, red or blue may also be seen.
- **D**iameter — There is change in size. The mole may be raised or flat, round or oval.

Other signs include a mole that scales, oozes, bleeds or changes in the way it feels. Some moles will become hard, lumpy, itchy, swollen or tender. Melanoma may also appear as a new mole.

OTHER SKIN CANCERS

Watch for skin irregularities that:

- Have a smooth, shiny or waxy surface
- Are small in size
- Bleed or become crusty
- Are flat or lumpy, red or pale

Prevention

The best approach to skin cancer is preventing it in the first place:

- Stay out of sun as much as possible, especially if you have fair skin, a history of sunburns or a current diagnosis of skin cancer.

- If you can't avoid sun exposure, wear protective clothing (hats and long sleeves) and gradually build up exposure to sunlight.

- Avoid or limit sunlight exposure between 11 a.m. and 1 p.m., when the sun's rays are the most direct.

- Some medications can greatly increase the likelihood of sunburn. Check all prescription and over-the-counter (OTC) medications for precautions about sun exposure.

- ALWAYS use sun block, even on overcast, cloudy days. Sunscreens are rated by a sun protection factor (SPF); the higher the SPF number, the greater the protection.

- Make sure children are adequately protected from the sun; exposure during childhood is a significant risk factor for developing skin cancer later in life.

- Check your skin regularly.

know
WHAT TO DO

Skin cancer
DO THESE APPLY:

- **Any skin lesion or growth that concerns you**
- **A change in the size, shape or feel of a mole**

YES

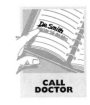

CALL DOCTOR

4

Eye pain

Burning, itching and discharge

Eye discomfort ranges from simple itching, which can be caused by a common cold or an allergic reaction, to pain which can be a symptom of much more serious eye disease.

Conjunctivitis (pinkeye) refers to an inflammation of the *conjunctiva* — the outermost membrane that covers the eye and inner part of the eyelid — and is the most common eye disease. Pinkeye can be caused by bacteria, viruses, allergies, pollution or other irritants such as cigarette smoke. The most common symptoms are redness of the whites of the eyes, scratchy or itchy eyes, tearing, swelling, yellow discharge that becomes crusty at night and sensitivity to light.

Newborns are susceptible to bacteria in the birth canal that can cause a type of conjunctivitis that must be treated immediately to prevent blindness.

In all cases of eye discomfort, it's best not to rub your eyes. This may aggravate symptoms and increase the chances of spreading a contagious infection to the other eye or to other people through personal contact. Most forms of eye discomfort respond well to self-care.

Prevention

There are some preventive measures that can reduce your risk of eye problems:

- Don't share towels.
- Never use anyone else's makeup.
- Discard your mascara after a couple of months.
- Wear goggles to protect your eyes against chlorinated swimming pools or airborne irritants such as chemicals or smoke.
- Air conditioning in your home and/or car can reduce allergens that cause eye discomfort.

What you can do

CONJUNCTIVITIS

- Avoid rubbing or touching your eyes.
- Wash your hands every time you touch your eyes. If you're around a child who has pinkeye, remember to wash your hands frequently with soap and water.
- Don't share washcloths or towels while infected with pinkeye.
- Change bed linens and pillowcases daily.
- Apply warm or cool compresses.
- If you wear contact lenses, remove them until the infection subsides.
- Over-the-counter (OTC) eye drops or boric acid washes can relieve itchiness.
- Antihistamines may help relieve allergic eye discomfort.

Final notes

Eye pain sometimes is caused by injury, infection or some other disease. Pain in both eyes when exposed to bright light is common with viral infections such as flu, and will disappear when the infection clears up. Injury to the eye by a foreign object also can cause pain. This type of eye pain should be treated by your doctor (see *Foreign Object In Eye*, p. 171).

see *Know What To Do*, p. 168

Eye pain

DO THESE APPLY:

- **Persistent eye pain**
- **Severe light sensitivity**
- **Vision impaired after wiping crusts from eye**
- **Pupils are different sizes**
- **Newborn has symptoms of conjunctivitis (irritated or itchy eyes, redness of white of eyes, tearing, yellow discharge, swelling, light sensitivity)**

YES

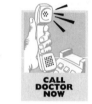

CALL DOCTOR NOW

NO

- **Watery drainage contains pus**
- **Symptoms spread from one eye to the other**
- **Symptoms don't improve after three to five days of self-care, or after a few days of prescribed treatment**
- **Symptoms begin to improve, then worsen**
- **Symptoms disappear completely for a short time but reappear in the same or other eye**

YES

CALL DOCTOR

NO

see *What You Can Do*
see *Styes*, p. 169

APPLY SELF-CARE

Styes

Painful, unsightly, but rarely harmful

Styes are caused by a bacterial infection of the tiny glands near the base of the eyelashes. They almost never result in damage to the eye or sight, and should not be confused with blocked tear ducts — which appear most commonly in infants as a bump along the side of the nose just below the inner corner of the eye.

A stye typically starts out looking like a pimple on the eyelid — a small, red, tender and swollen bump — and grows to full size over a day or so. The stye then fills with pus and ruptures within a few days. If the bacteria spread, more than one stye may occur. Styes can also form inside the eyelid, but this is less common.

What you can do

Wring out a clean cloth soaked in warm or hot water. Place it directly on the affected (closed) eye. For best results, do this three or four times a day for about 10 minutes each time. The stye will then rupture and drain, which usually occurs after about two days. Sometimes a stye may fade away without ever coming to a head and draining.

Since styes can be spread from one eye to another, and from one person to another through close contact, wash your hands frequently. Never pinch the stye to try to remove the pus, since this may also spread infection.

Final notes

Styes are common enough that many people can identify them on their own. Occasionally, they are confused with a *chalazion*, a swelling caused by a blocked gland within the eyelid. Unlike a stye, a chalazion is painless and is usually not helped by self-care.

A doctor may prescribe an antibiotic solution applied directly to the eyelid. Oral antibiotics are usually reserved for styes that do not respond to other treatment, are very large, or are located inside the eyelid. A particularly stubborn stye may need to be lanced and drained by a surgeon. Never try to do this on your own.

A stye can be extremely unpleasant because of its pain and appearance. Properly treated, it will disappear soon after it comes to a head and drains.

see *Know What To Do*, p. 170

4

Styes

DO THESE APPLY:

- **Swelling or redness spreading over the eye or tear duct**
- **Change in vision**
- **Eye pain or worsening symptoms**

YES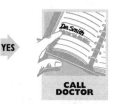

CALL DOCTOR NOW

NO

- **Stye keeps recurring**
- **Is under the eyelid**
- **Is still there after two days of self-care**
- **Crusty, yellow discharge on eyelid**

YES

CALL DOCTOR

NO

see *What You Can Do*

APPLY SELF-CARE

Foreign object in eye

Precautions, prevention and care

Tears and blinking are your natural defenses against sand, dust and other particles that enter the eye. But when something larger injures the eye, other steps are necessary to protect your vision and speed recovery.

Prevention

Nearly all eye injuries reported each year could have been prevented by wearing goggles or safety glasses during sports activities or while using tools (drills, hammers, grinders and saws) and heavy machinery. Other injuries could have been avoided by using common sense when handling fireworks, BB guns and other potential hazards.

What you can do

REMOVE ONLY THOSE OBJECTS FLOATING ON THE EYE'S SURFACE

Never rub the injured eye. Ask someone to help you remove the object from your eye, or use a mirror to locate it yourself. Sit in a well-lighted room, and use clean hands to pull the lower eyelid gently down while you look up. If you do not see the object, gently pull the upper lid out as you look down. Only attempt to remove foreign material if it is "floating." **Do not try to remove anything embedded in the eye. Seek emergency care.**

If you cannot readily see the object, grasp the lashes of your upper lid and pull down. Blink several times. This will sometimes remove small particles.

- Flush the eye with clean water by pressing the rim of a small glass against the eye socket and tilting your head back. Open and close the eye.

- If flushing with water is unsuccessful, moisten a cotton swab and gently lift off the object. Flush with water afterward.

- Do not use ointments or anesthetic drops on the eye.

4

HANDLING POSSIBLE COMPLICATIONS

- If a trip to the emergency room or doctor is necessary (see next page, *Know What To Do*), cover the eye with a sterile pad or clean cloth and keep it still. Close both eyes to prevent involuntary movement.
- If you can't close your eye, tape a paper cup over it.

Final notes

An object in the eye can scratch the *cornea* (the covering of the eye), and may cause significant vision loss. Your recovery will depend on how deep the object penetrates the eye, how quickly the injury is treated and whether an infection develops.

know
WHAT TO DO

Foreign object in eye
DO THESE APPLY:

- **Eye pain is severe**
- **Object is embedded, or on pupil or *iris* (colored part of eye)**
- **Object can't be located, but you felt something hit your eye**
- **Object can't be easily extracted**

YES →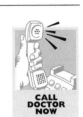

EMERGENCY ASSISTANCE

SEEK EMERGENCY CARE

—————————— **NO** ——————————

- **Pain and irritation continue for more than 24 hours, even if object was supposedly removed**

YES →

CALL DOCTOR NOW

—————————— **NO** ——————————

see *What You Can Do*

APPLY SELF-CARE

EAR/NOSE/THROAT

Sore throat

Common cold symptom, or more serious signal

A sore throat, or *pharyngitis,* is often the result of a viral or bacterial infection, although dry or polluted air, tobacco smoke or excessive alcohol use can also cause irritation. Typically, a sore throat is part of a cold or flu, or the result of postnasal drip from allergies, but in some cases it can be the symptom of a more serious condition that requires a doctor's care.

STREP THROAT

Strep throat is caused by an infection of the *streptococcal* bacteria, and untreated it can cause serious complications. Symptoms usually include severe sore throat, bright red throat, swollen tonsils and glands, and a fever higher than 101° F.

Strep usually targets children and may compound sore throat symptoms by making it difficult to open the mouth and causing the child to drool. It can spread rapidly, and some children may show no symptoms yet be carriers. When one child is diagnosed with strep, it's not uncommon for others in the family to come down with it as well.

Complications from strep may include inflammation of the kidneys and *rheumatic fever,* a painful joint disease that can also damage the heart. When a sore throat is prolonged, severe or is coupled with other symptoms, a throat culture is often taken to determine the cause. Antibiotics are the treatment for bacterial infections.

MONONUCLEOSIS

If an older child or adolescent has a severe sore throat combined with fatigue and a feeling of weakness, *infectious mononucleosis* (or mono) may be the cause. Mono is a viral infection which may bring about enlargement of the spleen but causes few complications. It rarely occurs in adults. A blood test will confirm the diagnosis, and treatment is limited to rest and plenty of fluids.

TONSILLITIS

Symptoms of *tonsillitis*, an inflammation and swelling of the *tonsils* (lymph tissues located on either side at the back of the throat) are similar to mononucleosis. Tonsillitis normally occurs in children and is usually caused by a viral infection. If the lymph nodes on the side of the neck are tender and swollen, and your child has foul-smelling breath, a bacterial infection may be the culprit.

In the past, doctors often removed the tonsils when a child had repeated tonsillitis or sore throats. Today the evidence suggests that the operation has no effect on the frequency of sore throats in most children.

INFLAMED ADENOIDS

Inflamed adenoids may trigger sore throats, as well, and they are common among children. Like the tonsils, the adenoids are lymph tissues in the back of the throat; however, adenoids are hard to see. Swollen adenoids can cause difficulty breathing, ear infections and sleep disturbances. Surgical removal of the adenoids, or an *adenoidectomy*, is rarely done and only when necessary.

What you can do

Because most sore throats are viral in origin, antibiotics are of little use. Time and patience are the greatest healers. Other tips:

- Use over-the-counter (OTC) pain relievers, such as aspirin, ibuprofen and acetaminophen (Tylenol), to ease the soreness. **NEVER give aspirin to children/teenagers. It can cause Reye's syndrome, a rare but often fatal condition.**
- Gargle with warm salt water (one teaspoon of salt added to eight ounces of water) several times a day.
- Use throat lozenges to soothe inflamed mucous membranes.
- Eat a soft or liquid diet to avoid irritating the throat.
- Drink plenty of liquids.

4

- Get plenty of rest.
- If you smoke, stop.

Final notes

While many adults suffer from an occasional sore throat while battling colds or the flu, children between the ages of 5 and 10 are very susceptible to the ailment. Fortunately, in most cases, the condition will disappear by itself in a week or so.

Sore throat
DO THESE APPLY:

- **Severe pain when swallowing**
- **Drooling**
- **Fever of 101° F or higher**
- **Severe malaise and sickly appearance**
- **Head is tilted toward one side, generally side with greatest pain**
- **Pus visible at back of throat**

YES → **CALL DOCTOR NOW**

NO

- **Diagnosed with sore throat and develop a rash, or a strawberry red tongue or throat**
- **Swollen glands in neck and fever lasting more than a few days**
- **Symptoms persist or worsen after a few days**
- **You have been exposed to strep throat**

YES → **CALL DOCTOR**

NO

see *What You Can Do*

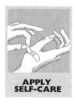

APPLY SELF-CARE

Laryngitis/ hoarseness

Finding your voice

Laryngitis is an inflammation of the *larynx* (voice box), which is located at the top of the windpipe. When the vocal cords, which are part of the larynx, become inflamed, they swell and cause hoarseness and distortion of the voice.

Laryngitis may be caused by illnesses such as the common cold, bronchitis or the flu, or by:

- Excessive talking, singing or shouting
- Allergies
- Inhaling irritating chemicals
- Excessive alcohol intake
- Heavy smoking

Note your symptoms

Laryngitis is usually identified by its primary symptom, hoarseness. Other symptoms can include loss of voice, tickling, rawness or pain in the throat, or a constant need to clear your throat.

What you can do

There is no specific medical treatment for laryngitis, but you may be able to relieve symptoms by:

- Resting your voice
- Inhaling steam (sit in the bathroom with the shower turned on hot to make steam)
- Drinking lots of liquids, especially warm, soothing ones
- Not smoking
- Gargling with warm salt water (one teaspoon of salt added to eight ounces of water) to soothe the throat
- Taking antihistamines to relieve symptoms caused by allergy

4

If laryngitis is caused by exposure to irritants, or alcoholism (see *Getting And Staying Healthy*, p. 372), the cause must be dealt with directly before the symptoms can be eliminated.

know
WHAT
TO DO

Laryngitis/hoarseness
DO THESE APPLY:

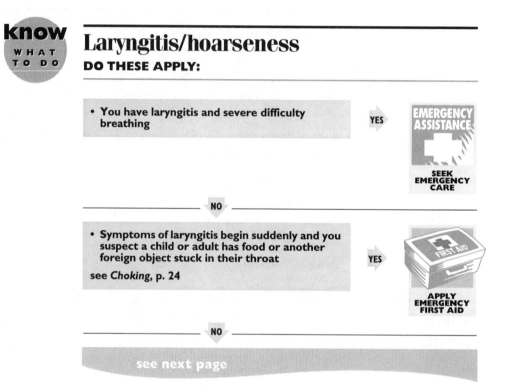

- **You have laryngitis and severe difficulty breathing**   **YES** → EMERGENCY ASSISTANCE / SEEK EMERGENCY CARE

NO

- **Symptoms of laryngitis begin suddenly and you suspect a child or adult has food or another foreign object stuck in their throat**
see *Choking*, p. 24   **YES** → FIRST AID / APPLY EMERGENCY FIRST AID

NO

see next page

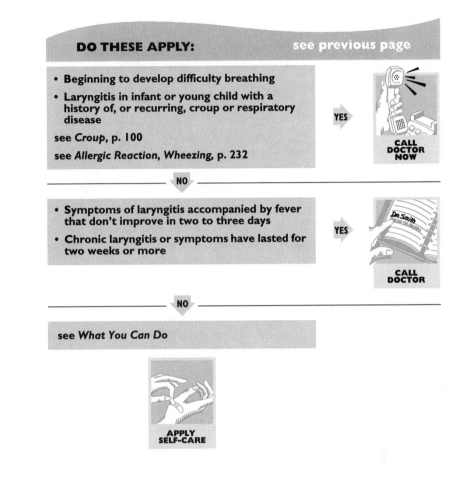

DO THESE APPLY: see previous page

- Beginning to develop difficulty breathing
- Laryngitis in infant or young child with a history of, or recurring, croup or respiratory disease

see *Croup*, p. 100

see *Allergic Reaction, Wheezing*, p. 232

YES → CALL DOCTOR NOW

NO

- Symptoms of laryngitis accompanied by fever that don't improve in two to three days
- Chronic laryngitis or symptoms have lasted for two weeks or more

YES → CALL DOCTOR

NO

see *What You Can Do*

APPLY SELF-CARE

4

Swollen glands

A sign of fighting infection

Lymph glands swell to help the body fight infection. Frequently, swollen glands mean there's an infection in the area of the body where the glands are located. For example, swollen neck glands frequently accompany sore throats and earaches. Lymph glands in the groin area sometimes swell when there is an infection in the feet, legs or genital region.

Swollen glands in the jaw can be a sign of *mumps* (see *Mumps*, p. 92) or a throat infection. Swollen glands behind the ears can be a sign of a scalp infection. If there is no scalp infection (see *Skin Symptoms*, p. 127), *German measles* (see *Rubella*, p. 86) or infectious *mononucleosis* (see *Sore Throat*, p. 174) could be the cause.

Glands become painful as a result of their rapid enlargement when they first begin to fight an infection. The pain usually goes away in a couple of days, but the lymph glands may stay enlarged for quite a while, sometimes several weeks.

On rare occasions, glands that have been enlarging over several weeks are a symptom of a serious underlying cause.

What you can do

If you have swollen glands and a sore throat that have been bothering you for less than two days, you can:

- Rest.
- Gargle with warm salt water (one teaspoon of salt added to eight ounces of water).
- Drink plenty of fluids.
- Suck on lozenges or hard candy.

Most swollen glands don't require any treatment because they are fighting an infection somewhere else in the body. An exception to this is if the gland itself develops a bacterial infection, making it red and tender. Sometimes a doctor will prescribe antibiotics to get rid of the bacteria causing the infection.

know
WHAT TO DO

Swollen glands

DO THESE APPLY:

- **Swollen glands and signs of infection in any of the extremities. Signs of infection are: redness around the area or red streaks leading away, swelling, warmth or tenderness, pus, fever of 101° F or higher, tender or swollen lymph nodes**
- **Swollen glands for more than two or three days, fever of 100.5° F, and a sore throat (with or without painful swallowing)**

YES▶

CALL DOCTOR NOW

NO▼

- **Swollen glands persist or have increased in size for two to three weeks**
- **Swollen glands accompanied by a possible scalp infection**
- **Swollen glands and rash**
- **Swollen glands and fever of 100.5° F for two to three days**

YES▶

CALL DOCTOR

NO▼

see *What You Can Do*

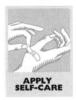

APPLY SELF-CARE

DIFFERENT SYMPTOMS?

see *Rubella*, p. 86; *Mumps*, p. 92; *Roseola*, p. 95;
Children's Ear Infections, p. 103;
Sore Throat, p. 174; *Earaches/Stuffiness*, p. 193

The common cold

Still outwitting modern medicine

A cold is a viral illness that can cause a sore throat, runny nose and other symptoms. Most colds are caused by *rhinoviruses* ("rhino" refers to the nose), which are transmitted through sneezes, coughs or handling virus-contaminated objects.

Prevention

Since there's no cure, avoiding the cold virus is the best way to beat the bug.

- Wash your hands frequently and teach your children to do the same.
- Avoid touching your eyes, nose or mouth after touching objects that could be contaminated with the cold virus, such as doorknobs or stair railings.

Note your symptoms

Cold symptoms develop suddenly within two to six days of exposure. A runny nose is a very common symptom. However, runny noses are also caused by hay fever or *allergic rhinitis* (see *Hay Fever,* p. 216), or by prolonged use of nose drops. Never use over-the-counter (OTC) nose drops for more than three consecutive days.

Foul-smelling, yellow or gray-green discharge coming from the nose usually indicates a bacterial infection. A foreign object in a nostril can prompt a runny nose, as well. In this case, the nose runs from one nostril and the discharge is foul-smelling (see *Object In The Nose,* p. 106).

The excess mucus produced by a runny nose can cause postnasal drip, which triggers a nighttime cough and can cause a sore throat. Ear or sinus infections may develop if mucus plugs up the eustachian tube between the nose and ear or the sinuses (see *Sinusitis,* p. 188; *Earaches/Stuffiness,* p. 193).

Other cold symptoms include:

- Scratchy or sore throat
- Sneezing
- Watery eyes

- Headache
- Swollen glands
- Cough that fails to bring up sputum
- Fever usually under 101° F in adults, but can climb to 103° F or 104° F in children (see *Fever*, p. 112)

A cold usually runs its course in five to seven days.

What you can do

SIMPLE STEPS TO RELIEF

- Get plenty of rest.
- Drink lots of fluids.
- Use a cool-mist vaporizer to relieve congestion. Change the water daily and rinse the vaporizer with a weak bleach and water solution.
- Ease nasal congestion in infants with a bulb syringe. Avoid excessive use to prevent damage to the inside of the nose.

MEDICATION CONSIDERATIONS

Over-the-counter (OTC) medications will not shorten the course of a cold, but they may offer temporary relief from some symptoms. All have side effects (see *Using Medications*, p. 362; *Home Pharmacy*, p. 364).

- Nose drops or nasal sprays are effective decongestants, but they can increase stuffiness if used for more than three consecutive days. Instead, substitute a homemade saline solution of one teaspoon of salt to a pint of water.
- Oral decongestants may act as stimulants and make you restless or unable to sleep. Often they are combined with antihistamines to lessen this side effect.
- Antihistamines appear to be more effective against allergy symptoms than cold-related complaints. They cause drowsiness, which can help you sleep. Never use antihistamines while driving or operating heavy machinery because of their tendency to cause drowsiness or dizziness.
- Pain relievers, such as aspirin, ibuprofen and acetaminophen (Tylenol), can lessen aches, pains and fevers. **NEVER give aspirin to children/teenagers. It can cause Reye's syndrome, a rare but often fatal condition.**

4

• Do not give nose drops, nasal spray or oral decongestants to children under 6 months of age. Relieve congestion with a homemade saline solution (see p. 183) or nasal syringe.

Final notes

In some cases, the common cold can lead to ear or sinus infections, laryngitis, bronchitis or pneumonia. Other conditions — such as strep throat, allergies and measles — produce symptoms which mimic a cold. Monitor the cold's progress — especially with children — and watch for high fevers, rashes, ear pain or breathing difficulty that can signal a more serious illness (see index).

know
WHAT
TO DO

Common cold
DO THESE APPLY:

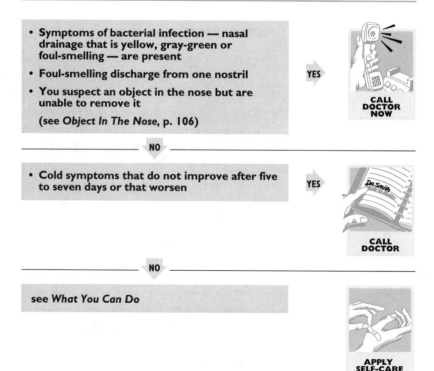

• **Symptoms of bacterial infection — nasal drainage that is yellow, gray-green or foul-smelling — are present**
• **Foul-smelling discharge from one nostril**
• **You suspect an object in the nose but are unable to remove it**
  (see *Object In The Nose*, p. 106)

YES ▸

CALL DOCTOR NOW

▾ **NO**

• **Cold symptoms that do not improve after five to seven days or that worsen**

YES ▸

CALL DOCTOR

▾ **NO**

see *What You Can Do*

APPLY SELF-CARE

Coughs

A natural defense mechanism

A cough is nature's way of sounding an alarm when something interferes with free breathing. It's a natural reflex designed to clear your breathing tubes of mucus and foreign particles.

Note your symptoms

Coughs are usually referred to as "productive" or "nonproductive." A productive cough jars loose phlegm or pus and helps expel it from the body. You'll probably be advised to let a productive cough do its work and avoid cough suppressants. A nonproductive cough is dry or hacking, and you may need to take steps to quiet it. Learning to spot a cough's characteristics can help you pinpoint the appropriate steps for relief.

Some common causes for dry, nonproductive coughs are dry air, smoking and postnasal drip. Productive coughs, meanwhile, may signal viral or bacterial infections. Mucus is usually yellow or white with a viral infection, but it can be yellow, gray-green or rust-colored and contain pus with a bacterial infection. Bacterial infections usually require antibiotics.

Coughs in infants are very unusual and can suggest a serious problem. In older infants and young children, a cough may signal a foreign object lodged in the throat. A youngster's barking cough may mean croup (see *Croup*, p. 100).

What you can do

- Drink lots of water to loosen phlegm and soothe your irritated throat.
- Use a cool-mist vaporizer to increase humidity.
- Use throat lozenges or hard candies to relieve the "tickle" and throat irritation.
- If postnasal drip is causing the dry, hacking cough, try an over-the-counter (OTC) decongestant. Avoid medications with antihistamines, which will thicken the secretions you are trying to dislodge.

4

- Try a nonprescription cough medication containing *guaifenesin*, which can thin secretions. Over-the-counter (OTC) cough suppressants with *dextromethorphan* may help quiet the cough at night so you can get some rest (see *Home Pharmacy*, p. 364).

- Use pillows to elevate your head at night.

- If you smoke, stop.

Final notes

Hiccups may seem related to coughs, but they're actually caused by irregular contractions of the diaphragm. Home remedies abound for this annoying reflex action. One example is simply holding your breath.

Coughs

DO THESE APPLY:

- Hard cough began suddenly and without other symptoms, especially in a child who might have inhaled an object
- In a child, cough is combined with rapid, difficult breathing or wheezing

YES ▶

EMERGENCY ASSISTANCE

SEEK EMERGENCY CARE

--- NO ---

- Child is less than 3 months old
- Mucus expelled is yellow, gray-green or rust-colored, or foul-smelling

YES ▶

CALL DOCTOR NOW

--- NO ---

- Fever for more than four days
- Cough lingers more than seven to 10 days after other symptoms have cleared
- Coughing is causing you to become increasingly fatigued

YES ▶

CALL DOCTOR

--- NO ---

see *What You Can Do*

APPLY SELF-CARE

Sinusitis

It's all in your head

Sinusitis is an inflammation of the *sinuses*, the four pairs of empty chambers in the facial bones around the nose and eyes. These chambers are located near the cheekbones, above the eyebrows, behind or between the eyes and near the temples. Inflammation can be caused by viral, bacterial or fungal infection, or by allergies.

The condition is usually brought on by an upper respiratory tract infection, hay fever (see *Hay Fever*, p. 216) or a *deviated septum* (a deformity in the structure between the nostrils that divides the inside of the nose into right and left sides). About 25% of chronic sinusitis in the area near the cheekbones is related to dental infections (see *Dental Care*, p. 204).

Note your symptoms

- Tenderness and swelling over the area involved
- Pain around the eyes or cheeks
- Difficulty breathing through the nose
- Inside of nose is red and swollen
- Yellow or gray-green nasal discharge
- General feeling of illness
- Fever may or may not be present

What you can do

- Inhaling steam helps promote drainage. Try sitting in a steamy bathroom.

- Stay indoors and keep rooms at an even temperature.

- Drink plenty of fluids (a glass of water or juice every one to two hours).

- Nasal sprays such as phenylephrine 0.25% may be effective, but they should not be used for more than three consecutive days.

- Over-the-counter (OTC) decongestants may help open the nasal passages and cause drainage of the sinuses.

- Hot and cold compresses applied to the forehead and cheeks (apply them alternately, one minute each, for 10 minutes) may aid sinus drainage.

- Increasing home humidity may help.

Anyone with a history of recurring sinusitis should use self-care treatment at the first sign of a cold or other respiratory tract infection or when they experience an allergic reaction.

A doctor may prescribe antibiotics to treat chronic sinusitis or sinusitis caused by a bacterial infection. On rare occasions, surgical repair of the sinuses may be necessary.

see *Know What To Do*, p. 190

Sinusitis

DO THESE APPLY:

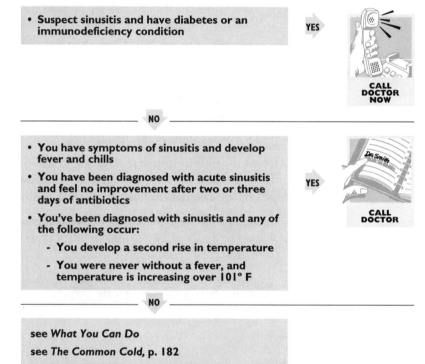

- Suspect sinusitis and have diabetes or an immunodeficiency condition

    YES → **CALL DOCTOR NOW**

_____ NO _____

- You have symptoms of sinusitis and develop fever and chills

- You have been diagnosed with acute sinusitis and feel no improvement after two or three days of antibiotics

- You've been diagnosed with sinusitis and any of the following occur:

    - You develop a second rise in temperature

    - You were never without a fever, and temperature is increasing over 101° F

    YES → **CALL DOCTOR**

_____ NO _____

see *What You Can Do*

see *The Common Cold*, p. 182

see *Hay Fever*, p. 216

APPLY SELF-CARE

Nosebleeds

Self-care almost always works

Nosebleeds are usually messier and more embarrassing than they are serious, and can almost always be stopped with self-care. Nosebleeds are usually caused by trauma to the nose or by anything that irritates normal tissue integrity, such as dry air, low humidity, allergies, picking the nose or blowing the nose during a cold.

Prevention

Frequently, nosebleeds are related to the common cold — the blood vessels in the nose are irritated by either a virus or constant nose blowing. If this is the case, treating cold symptoms reduces the probability of having more nosebleeds.

Nosebleeds tend to occur more often in the winter when people spend more time indoors where the air is dry and heated. Turning the heat down and using a cool-mist vaporizer to put moisture back into the air sometimes brings relief from nosebleeds.

Finding the cause of recurring nosebleeds is, of course, the first step in preventing them.

What you can do

When you have a nosebleed:

- Sit in a chair, keeping your head level rather than tilted back. This prevents the blood from running down your throat.
- Squeeze the nostrils shut between your thumb and forefinger.
- Breathe through your mouth and apply pressure for 10 full minutes without letting go of your nose.
- Cold compresses or ice packs applied to the bridge of the nose may also help. For protection, place a washcloth between bare skin and ice.
- If the bleeding hasn't stopped, apply pressure for another 10 minutes. This method almost always works if enough time is allowed for the bleeding to stop.

When the bleeding stops, try to remain quiet for a few hours. Don't blow your nose, laugh or talk loudly.

see *Know What To Do*, p. 192

Nosebleeds

DO THESE APPLY:

• **Nosebleed is accompanied by suspected nose fracture (deformity is seen in the profile of the nose)**

• **Bleeding is heavy and won't stop with self-care**

YES →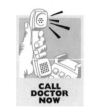
CALL DOCTOR NOW

NO

• **Nosebleeds are recurring and cause is undetermined**

YES →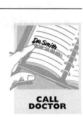
CALL DOCTOR

NO

see *What You Can Do*

see *The Common Cold,* p. 182

APPLY SELF-CARE

EARACHES/STUFFINESS

When fluid accumulates in the *middle ear* (that part of the ear behind the eardrum) pressure builds up and causes pain. Problems are most common among children (see *Children's Ear Infections,* p. 103 and *Ear Discharge,* p. 197), but they can also affect adults.

Middle ear infection

Persistent ear pain is a symptom

Middle ear infections (*otitis media*) usually occur as a complication of an upper respiratory infection (see index for *Colds, Hay Fever* and *Sinusitis*), when the tubes between the ear and the throat (*eustachian tubes*) swell and close. Fluid and mucus gather in the middle ear and bacteria breed.

The hallmark symptom of otitis media — persistent ear pain — may be accompanied by decreased hearing, a ringing or sense of fullness in the ear, fever, headache, dizziness and runny nose.

What you can do

Otitis media requires a visit to your doctor, who will probably prescribe antibiotic treatment and possibly a decongestant.

Self-care includes:

- Getting plenty of rest
- Increasing consumption of clear fluids
- Placing a warm washcloth, water bottle or heating pad (set on low) directly on the affected ear
- Blowing your nose gently, with your mouth open
- Using a cool-mist vaporizer to moisturize the air and help control levels of mucus

- Taking acetaminophen (Tylenol), ibuprofen or aspirin to relieve discomfort; antihistamines, decongestants or nose drops may help decrease the amount of nasal secretion and shrink mucous membranes. **NEVER give aspirin to children/teenagers. It can cause Reye's syndrome, a rare but often fatal condition.**

NOTE: Do not insert **any** type of object in the ear to relieve itching or pain.

see *Know What To Do*, p. 196

Ruptured eardrum

Requires a visit to the doctor

Pressure building up in the middle ear, blows to the ear, or sharp objects can cause the eardrum to rupture. Symptoms may include mild to severe ear pain, partial temporary hearing loss, and a white to yellowish discharge from the ear (see *Ear Discharge*, p. 197).

See a doctor promptly; antibiotics may be prescribed to prevent or treat an infection in the middle ear.

A one-time rupture is not serious (repeated eardrum ruptures may cause hearing loss). The eardrum usually heals within two months.

What you can do

Pain can be relieved by using over-the-counter (OTC) pain relievers and a heating pad set on low. Hearing almost always returns to normal after the eardrum heals.

see *Know What To Do*, p. 196

Fluid in middle ear

Usually clears up on its own

Serous otitis media results when fluid collects in the middle ear, either from a previous infection or ongoing irritations such as allergies. An infection is not necessarily associated with this condition but can occur if bacteria build up. Symptoms may include temporary hearing loss and a feeling of stuffiness or sensitivity in the ear.

What you can do

Most cases of serous otitis media clear up in about a week. Chewing gum and swallowing may help open the eustachian tube, and decongestants or antihistamines may provide additional relief.

If the problem does not clear up with self-care, a doctor may prescribe a higher dose of decongestant or use a device to force air into the eustachian tube and middle ear. If a bacterial infection is involved, antibiotics may be prescribed.

see *Know What To Do*, p. 196

Barotitis

That blocked-up feeling in the ears

"Airplane ears" (or *barotitis*) usually occurs as a result of air pressure changes — driving in the mountains, flying in an airplane — or when you have a cold or stuffy nose. This results in a blocked-up feeling in the ears.

What you can do

- Yawning, swallowing, chewing gum or gently blowing through your nose — while holding your nose shut and closing your mouth — may solve the problem. Using decongestant nasal sprays 30 minutes before the airplane begins to land can also help.
- For infants, offer a bottle or let them nurse to clear ears.

know
WHAT
TO DO

Earaches/stuffiness
DO THESE APPLY:

- **Ear pain accompanied by headache, fever and stiff neck**

  see *Meningitis*, p. 271

YES

SEEK
EMERGENCY
CARE

—————————— NO ——————————

- **White-to-yellowish or foul-smelling ear discharge**

  see *Ear Discharge*, p. 197

- **Sudden loss of hearing**

YES

CALL
DOCTOR
NOW

—————————— NO ——————————

- **Ear infection is suspected**
- **Acute ear pain lasts more than an hour**
- **Any earache lasting longer than 12 - 24 hours**
- **Symptoms of barotitis do not improve after taking a decongestant for a day or two**
- **Symptoms increase — or fail to improve — after two or three days of antibiotic treatment**
- **Stuffy ears or hearing loss persists, without other symptoms, more than 10 days after cold clears up**

YES

CALL
DOCTOR

—————————— NO ——————————

see *What You Can Do*

see *Children's Ear Infections*, p. 103

APPLY
SELF-CARE

EAR DISCHARGE

Ear discharge is usually just ear wax but can also be the result of a minor infection or a ruptured eardrum.

Ear wax

It almost never causes problems

The purpose of ear wax is to protect the ear and keep it clean. The wax is normally in a liquid form and will drain by itself. Ear wax almost never causes problems unless you try to "clean" your ears using a cotton swab or some other instrument, which can pack the ear wax down tightly. If the ear wax builds up, it can become crusty and black, sometimes causing a stuffy feeling and hearing loss.

Ear wax usually will not cause pain or a fever. If you experience these symptoms, suspect an ear infection (see *Earaches/Stuffiness*, p. 193).

Prevention

In most cases, taking warm showers or washing the outside of the ears with a washcloth and warm water provides enough vapor to prevent the buildup of wax.

Children normally have more ear wax than adults. The ears should be left alone unless the ear wax is causing some problem, like a ringing in the ears or a hearing loss.

What you can do

Normally, packed-down ear wax can be removed by gently flushing the ear with warm water using a syringe (available at drugstores). Always use water that is as close to body temperature as possible. Using cold water can result in dizziness and vomiting.

Wax softeners such as olive oil, Debrox or Cerumenex, also can be used. Follow instructions carefully for commercial softening products.

Never put anything into the ear if you think the eardrum might be ruptured.

see *Know What To Do*, p. 199

4

RUPTURED EARDRUM

If you've recently had a cold with ear pain and congestion, and then notice ear discharge (even on your pillow), contact your doctor. Infections, blows to the head or inserting sharp objects into the ear can rupture the eardrum (see *Ruptured Eardrum*, p. 194).

Swimmer's ear

Feels like your ear is full of water

Swimmer's ear (*otitis externa*) is a persistent irritation and inflammation of the outer ear canal that occurs after swimming, or after repeated attempts are made to clean ear wax from the ear.

Symptoms include tenderness and a feeling of fullness (like the ear is full of water), itching, burning and pain when the outer ear is tugged. More serious cases will cause redness of the ear canal; a crusty, pus-filled discharge; and possibly some hearing loss.

Prevention

The key is to dry the ears immediately after swimming or showering by shaking the head to remove trapped water. Use the twisted corners of a facial tissue to dry each ear. Tip your head to the left as you dry the left ear, and repeat for your right.

Swim-team members or others who spend a lot of time in water can take over-the-counter (OTC) or prescription ear drops to change the acid/alkali level in the ear canal and potentially prevent swimmer's ear.

What you can do

- Look in the ear with a light to make sure there isn't an object or insect in the ear.

- Try rinsing the affected ear with a homemade solution (half warm water, half white vinegar). Gently insert solution into ear with a bulb syringe.

- Use swimmer's ear drops. Have the affected person lie down, ear facing up. Place over-the-counter (OTC) drops (or a few drops of rubbing alcohol mixed with white vinegar) on the canal wall in small quantities, so air can escape. If air gets trapped, it will keep the solution from penetrating. Wiggle the ear to avoid this problem.

- Use a heating pad set on low and over-the-counter (OTC) pain relievers to ease discomfort. **NEVER give aspirin to children/ teenagers. It can cause Reye's syndrome, a rare but often fatal condition.**

- Try to keep the ear as dry as possible until the infection subsides.

Final notes

As the old saying goes, don't put anything smaller than your elbow in your ear. Inserting hairpins or other instruments can be dangerous because injury to the eardrum can result. Cotton swabs generally pack down ear wax instead of getting it out of the ear and push foreign bodies farther into the ear.

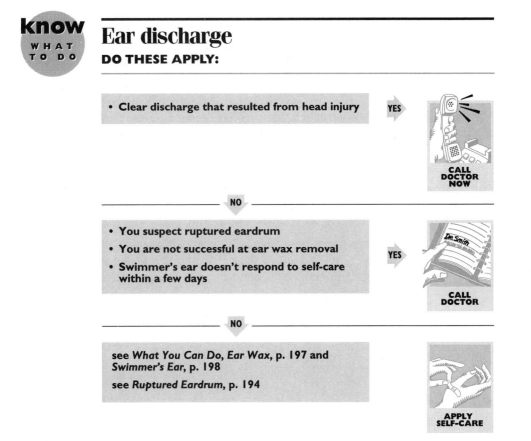

know
WHAT
TO DO

Ear discharge
DO THESE APPLY:

- **Clear discharge that resulted from head injury**   YES →

**CALL
DOCTOR
NOW**

NO

- **You suspect ruptured eardrum**
- **You are not successful at ear wax removal**   YES →
- **Swimmer's ear doesn't respond to self-care within a few days**

**CALL
DOCTOR**

NO

see *What You Can Do, Ear Wax*, p. 197 and *Swimmer's Ear*, p. 198

see *Ruptured Eardrum*, p. 194

**APPLY
SELF-CARE**

4

MOUTH CONCERNS

Oral herpes

Causes cold sores and fever blisters

Oral herpes is a common viral infection characterized by small, fluid-filled sores on the skin and mucous membranes of the mouth. This herpes simplex type 1 virus is not the same as — but is related to — herpes simplex type 2, which causes *genital herpes*.

About 90% of Americans are infected with oral herpes by the age of 5. Following the initial infection, the virus remains dormant with new episodes recurring at different frequencies for different people. New outbreaks can be triggered by a variety of factors including dental treatment, sunburn, food allergies, anxiety, menstruation, fever-producing illness or a damaged immune system.

Prevention

The virus is very contagious and can be transmitted through personal contact or contact with contaminated objects such as kitchen utensils, razors or towels. If you have an active infection, avoid close physical contact with others and do not share personal items.

What you can do

- Salves can relieve pain, but are not effective in all cases. Try various methods, such as over-the-counter (OTC) oral and topical analgesics. Use what works best for you.
- Acyclovir (Zovirax) is an antiviral agent that may speed healing if applied during the initial outbreak. Oral acyclovir is sometimes prescribed for frequent or severe outbreaks.

Attacks of oral herpes usually go away, with or without treatment, within seven days and have no lasting complications.

see *Know What To Do*, p. 203

Canker sores

Also known as aphthous stomatitis

The canker sore is a painful ulcer that develops on the gums, tongue or inside the mouth. The cause is unknown but any of the following increase the likelihood of getting one: viruses; allergies; gastrointestinal disease; immune reactions; deficiencies of iron, B₁₂ or folic acid; and stress and trauma to the inside of the mouth.

What you can do

There's no known way to prevent canker sores, but nonprescription topical anesthetic gels or rinses (such as 2% lidocaine) will lessen the pain. A dental protective paste, such as Orabase, prevents irritation of the sores.

see *Know What To Do*, p. 203

Thrush

An infection of the mouth and throat

Thrush, or *oral candidiasis*, is a fungal yeast infection that causes painful, creamy-white sore patches in the mouth or throat. Eating or brushing your teeth can cause the patches to be scraped off, causing bleeding.

In adults, thrush may signify that a more serious underlying condition exists. Occasionally, it may affect the entire body. This life-threatening infection is extremely rare except in those who already are debilitated by other conditions, such as AIDS or immunosuppressive therapy.

Thrush is common in infants and children and will often disappear without treatment. In infants, obvious discomfort while feeding or an unwillingness to eat may indicate thrush.

What you can do

Although thrush will often disappear on its own, an antifungal medication will usually speed healing. Nystatin, in liquid or tablets, may be recommended by your doctor. With treatment, symptoms usually disappear within seven to 10 days.

A diet of soft foods may lessen discomfort until the symptoms are gone.

see *Know What To Do*, p. 203

Coxsackie Virus

And other causes of mouth sores

Coxsackie virus, or *hand-foot-mouth syndrome*, can also cause mouth sores in children. The virus, which usually includes spots on the hands and feet, goes away by itself. The symptoms are mild and the child generally feels well.

The goals for treatment are to relieve pain caused by the mouth sores and maintain an adequate fluid intake — mouth sores can often interfere with eating or drinking. A child can go several days without taking a full meal, but it is very important to get enough liquid. Try offering drinks that soothe a tender mouth, such as cold liquids, Popsicles or frozen juices.

Mouth sores
DO THESE APPLY:

- **An undiagnosed mouth sore persists for two weeks**
- **Suspect medication may be causing mouth sores**
- **Pregnant**
- **Painful outbreak of ulcers on gums, tongue or inside of mouth, especially with large or multiple lesions (suggestive of canker sores)**
- **Frequent or severe cold sores**
- **Creamy-white sore patches inside mouth, on tongue or in throat (suggestive of thrush)**
- **You are being treated for thrush and signs and symptoms persist for more than 10 days**

YES → **CALL DOCTOR**

NO

see *What You Can Do*

see *Coxsackie Virus*, p. 202

see *Oral Herpes*, p. 200

see *Canker Sores*, p. 201

APPLY SELF-CARE

Dental care

Giving your teeth a good, long life

Prevention. That's the key word in dental care — taking care of your teeth now to avoid future problems. Since teeth are living organisms, they are subject to damage from the foods we eat, especially those containing sugar. Bacteria that are not removed from the teeth by brushing or flossing become a sticky, colorless film called *plaque*. Food particles, especially sugar, stick to plaque and produce acid. This acid damages tooth enamel. When this damage, or decay, spreads down the root canal to the nerve, it causes pain and inflammation. In other words: a toothache.

Another problem caused by an accumulation of plaque is gum disease, or *gingivitis*. It is an inflammation of the gums that can cause redness, discomfort, swelling, watery discharge and bleeding when you brush or chew. Gingivitis also causes the gums to become deformed, with the crevice between the gums and teeth deepening and forming pockets. In severe cases, this can result in tooth loss.

Prevention

Most dental problems can be prevented by good self-care and regular visits to the dentist. With proper care and injury prevention, we can expect to keep our teeth for life, unlike our parents' and grandparents' generations. Here are some ways to keep teeth and gums healthy.

REGULAR CHECKUPS

Have teeth professionally cleaned every six to 12 months, beginning at about age 3. Regular dental checkups can provide early detection of gingivitis, cavities and other problems, making treatment easier.

BRUSHING

Brush teeth thoroughly twice a day, especially after eating when possible. The goal is to remove plaque from all surfaces of the teeth. Children over 3 years old and adults should use a soft-bristle toothbrush with rounded tips, and replace it every three to four months. Use a small amount (pea size) of fluoride toothpaste.

Water piks and electric toothbrushes are controversial, but they may help some people clean hard-to-reach areas. Check with your dentist regarding what's best for you.

The formation of *tartar*, mineral deposits that get trapped on the teeth by plaque, can be slowed by tartar-control toothpastes.

Be sure to brush the tongue as well as the teeth. Plaque on the tongue can cause bad breath. Also, since you can actually harm your gums by brushing too hard or in the wrong direction, consult your dentist on the best brushing procedures.

FLOSSING

Daily flossing is the best way to prevent gum disease between teeth. The purpose is to scrape off the plaque that forms between the teeth and just under the gum line.

The various types of dental floss (waxed, unwaxed, extra fine, flossing tape and flossing ribbons) each have advantages. Select the type that works best on your teeth.

The most important aspect of flossing is to curve the floss around the tooth being cleaned and slide it under the gum line. With both fingers holding the floss against the tooth, move the floss up and down several times to scrape off the plaque.

Flossing should be started with children as soon as they have teeth that touch each other. A child usually can't floss their own teeth until around the age of 8. Using a flossing tool can be helpful in doing a good job in a small mouth.

DISCLOSING TABLETS

Disclosing tablets are small, chewable tablets that can be found at most drugstores. Chew the tablet and swish with water. The tablet will color any plaque that remains on the teeth. By using a flashlight and dental mirror, you can see where you've been missing the plaque with your regular brushing and flossing routines. This is especially helpful (and fun) for children in reinforcing good dental habits.

4

FLUORIDE

Fluoride is a mineral found in most food and water supplies that strengthens tooth enamel and lowers the risk of tooth decay. In many areas of the country, fluoride is added to the water because the natural levels of fluoride are too low to protect teeth.

Infants and children in low-fluoride areas can be given fluoride supplements in the form of tablets or drops. Fluoride toothpastes, rinses or topical applications are also beneficial.

SEALANTS

Sealants are a plastic coating usually applied to children's back teeth. They protect the *molars* (the larger chewing teeth at the back of the mouth) from developing decay. By using sealants and fluoride, it is possible for children to grow up without cavities.

What you can do

If you have a toothache, taking aspirin, ibuprofen or acetaminophen (Tylenol) may lessen the pain while a dental appointment is being made. **NEVER give aspirin to children/teenagers. It can cause Reye's syndrome, a rare but often fatal condition.**

Final notes

Do not put infants or young children to bed with a bottle filled with juice, sugar water, milk or formula. These liquids pool around teeth and can cause serious tooth decay called *bottle mouth*.

see *Know What To Do*, p. 209

see *Accidental Tooth Loss*, p. 64

Temporomandibular joint syndrome (TMJ)

When your jaw is "on the blink"

This is a condition in which jaw movement is abnormal. The temporomandibular joint attaches the jaw to the skull. Abnormalities and inflammation of this joint can produce pain, difficulty in opening and closing your mouth, clicking or grinding sounds while chewing, ringing in the ears and occasionally hearing loss.

Causes of TMJ include the failure of the jaw to close properly, poorly fitting dentures, arthritis, trauma from fractures or dislocations of the jaw, stress-induced muscle tension and repetitive tooth grinding.

Note your symptoms

Depending on the underlying cause, symptoms can vary with each individual. Common symptoms include:

- Pain over the TMJ area (on either side of the face, in front of the ears)

- Dull ear pain without fever

- Dull headaches

- Grinding, clicking or popping sounds

- Ringing in the ears

- Limited mouth opening

Some sufferers of TMJ may suddenly dislocate their jaw, causing pain and making it impossible to close the mouth after yawning or while chewing.

Other causes of jaw pain include *angina pectoris* (pain from coronary artery disease) and sinus and ear infections (see index for these topics).

What you can do

- Over-the-counter (OTC) anti-inflammatory medications may relieve pain.

- Rest the jaw, keeping teeth apart and lips closed.

- Avoid foods that are hard to chew.

- Avoid chewing gum, tooth grinding and other activities that cause repetitive movements of the jaw.

- Applying moist heat to the jaw for 20 minutes three times a day may help (unless TMJ is the result of injury).

- Use ice packs on the joint for five to eight minutes three times a day. For protection, place a washcloth between bare skin and ice.

- When pain has stopped, gentle exercises — opening and closing the mouth — can improve jaw muscle strength and flexibility.

Dental care/TMJ

DO THESE APPLY:

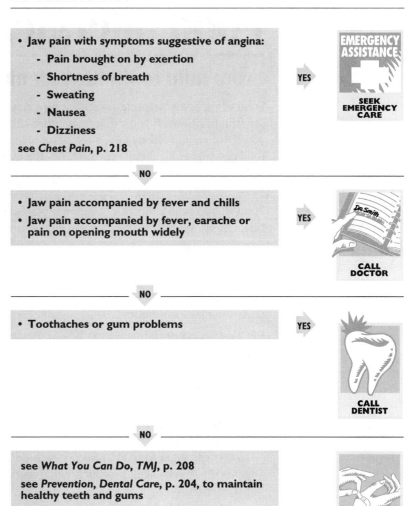

- Jaw pain with symptoms suggestive of angina:
    - Pain brought on by exertion
    - Shortness of breath
    - Sweating
    - Nausea
    - Dizziness

see *Chest Pain*, p. 218

YES → **EMERGENCY ASSISTANCE** — **SEEK EMERGENCY CARE**

— NO —

- Jaw pain accompanied by fever and chills
- Jaw pain accompanied by fever, earache or pain on opening mouth widely

YES → **CALL DOCTOR**

— NO —

- Toothaches or gum problems

YES → **CALL DENTIST**

— NO —

see *What You Can Do, TMJ*, p. 208

see *Prevention, Dental Care*, p. 204, to maintain healthy teeth and gums

APPLY SELF-CARE

ALLERGIES

Food allergies

From mild to life-threatening

Food allergies are suspected when eating a certain food triggers adverse physical reactions. If you suffer from other allergies, such as hay fever, you are often more likely to be affected (see *Hay Fever*, p. 216). Nearly any food can trigger an allergic reaction, but the most common culprits are seafood, eggs, nuts and seeds.

Note your symptoms

Food allergies can prompt a wide range of reactions, in some cases life-threatening. Symptoms appear soon after eating and may include:

- Runny nose

- Vomiting and stomach cramps

- Eczema (see *Eczema*, p. 130)

- Asthma (see *Asthma*, p. 213)

- Constriction or tightening of chest, difficulty breathing, fever, violent coughing and an irregular pulse. This is very likely a severe *anaphylactic* reaction and can quickly lead to death. **Seek emergency care immediately.**

- Infants usually experience few allergy symptoms; eczema and/or stomach upset are the primary clues. If vomiting and diarrhea occur after drinking milk, the problem may actually be an intolerance to *lactose,* the sugar found in milk. These food allergy symptoms generally fade by age 12 months, while respiratory symptoms may persist.

What you can do

IF YOU KNOW WHAT FOODS PRODUCE REACTIONS

- Avoid foods that produce allergic symptoms. Make sure friends and relatives know of your allergies so you are not exposed to these foods without knowing it when dining in their homes.

- Ask about the ingredients in foods when eating out.
- Be aware that foods can contain unexpected ingredients.
- If you are at risk for anaphylactic reactions, consider obtaining an anaphylactic kit to inject medication if necessary. Your doctor can provide you with a prescription.
- Consider wearing a medical-alert bracelet to inform others of your allergy.

IF YOU DON'T KNOW WHAT CAUSES YOUR REACTIONS

- Keep a food diary and list symptoms you experience after eating.
- Try eliminating foods from your diet one at a time, and note any reactions.
- Introduce new foods to young children one at a time.

Final notes

Food allergy reactions generally become more acute each time the food is eaten, making it even more important to identify foods that cause severe reactions.

see *Know What To Do*, p. 212

know
WHAT
TO DO

Food allergies
DO THESE APPLY:

- **Sudden and severe hives**
- **Lips, mouth, face or neck swollen**
- **Mouth or throat tingles**
- **Stomach is distended**
- **Difficulty breathing**
- **Cyanosis (blue- or purple-tinged skin)**
- **Convulsions**
- **Loss of consciousness**
  see *Unconsciousness*, p. 40

YES
SEEK EMERGENCY CARE

NO

- **Slight fever**
- **Reddened skin, itching or hives**
- **Intestinal spasms, tingling and swelling of mouth, throat, lips**
- **Increased irritability**

YES
CALL DOCTOR NOW

NO

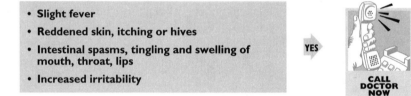

- **Certain foods seem to trigger reaction**

YES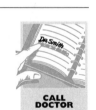
CALL DOCTOR

NO

see *What You Can Do*

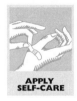
APPLY SELF-CARE

Asthma

Self-care can make a big difference

Asthma is an allergic disease that inflames and constricts the airways to the lungs and causes coughing, wheezing, chest pain and an increased production of mucus. Frequently, an asthma attack gives the feeling of suffocation or even panic.

About half of all asthma cases develop before the age of 10, and about one-third develop before age 40. In childhood, boys are twice as likely to suffer from asthma as girls, but after adolescence it's about the same for both sexes. Recent evidence shows that more than half of all asthmatic children will never have an asthma attack as adults, and only 10% will suffer occasional attacks as adults.

If you have allergies, you're particularly susceptible to asthma. Most people with asthma are sensitive to dust, animal dander, pollen, mold and other common allergens. If you're like most people with asthma, appropriate care and drug therapy can help you lead a normal, active life. There is no routine screening to detect the likelihood of developing asthma.

Prevention

If you've experienced asthma attacks, these are some steps you can take to reduce the number and severity of attacks:

- Eliminate or reduce exposure to "triggers" that cause attacks, such as cigarette smoke, pollen, dust and other irritants.

- If pollen triggers attacks, stay inside as much as possible during periods of high pollen count — preferably an inside environment with filtered air.

- Remove the carpets in your home, and at work if possible, to decrease attacks. Dust mites, which often trigger attacks, thrive in carpeting.

- Enclose your mattress in a plastic zipper bag (make sure there are no openings or tears in it) to reduce your exposure to potential allergens.

- Drink plenty of fluids, which may loosen mucus in your lungs and make breathing easier.

- If your doctor has given you an acute-care regimen and you begin to have an attack, implement the measures immediately. The key to managing an asthma attack is to prevent it from getting out of control.

- Keep a record of daily treatment, acute-care regimen, and pertinent information about symptoms, treatment and your response to treatment.

What you can do

Self-evaluation and self-care are the most important things you can do to control asthma attacks. Discuss a self-care plan with your doctor that includes:

- Daily or routine drug therapy

- Ways to monitor symptoms

- What medications to take when an attack begins

- When to seek medical or emergency care

Final notes

Your doctor will diagnose asthma by taking your medical history and performing a physical examination. In some cases, tests of lung function and chest x-rays also may be used to confirm the diagnosis.

Asthma drugs are often administered using a *metered dose inhaler* (MDI). This tubular device propels small particles of drug through the mouth into the lungs. If you have difficulty using an MDI, your doctor may recommend modifications for proper drug treatment.

know
WHAT TO DO

Asthma
DO THESE APPLY:

- **Significant respiratory distress — such as rapid breathing or difficulty breathing and/or bluish discoloration to the skin**
- **Confusion or lethargy**
- **Sharp chest pains**
- **Asthma attack is out of control**

YES → **EMERGENCY ASSISTANCE**
SEEK EMERGENCY CARE

NO

- **Difficulty breathing**
- **Increased coughing**
- **Little relief after following prescribed regimen for acute attacks**
- **Attack seems to be getting out of control**

YES → **CALL DOCTOR NOW**

NO

- **You have asthma and do not have a self-care plan that includes what to do when attack begins**
- **You have not been diagnosed with asthma but have noticed:**
  - **Dry cough with exercise and/or at night**
  - **Difficulty breathing, tight chest, wheezing**

YES → **CALL DOCTOR**

NO

see *What You Can Do*

APPLY SELF-CARE

4

Hay fever

To everything there is a season

Hay fever sufferers can blame pollen for the sneezing, watery eyes and runny nose that mark this common allergy. Some form of pollen is almost always in the air, whether from trees in the spring, summer grass or fall ragweed. The severity of your symptoms can depend on the time of year and the amount of airborne pollen on a particular day.

Note your symptoms

Hay fever occurs when your body's antibodies react to pollen and prompt the release of *histamine*. Histamine inflames the lining of nasal passages and causes sneezing, itching and watery eyes. Headaches, irritability and insomnia are possible, too.

Hay fever can be confused with the common cold, but you can suspect you have allergies if your symptoms last for long periods of time and return during the same season each year. If hay fever runs in your family, chances are your sneezes are based on allergies, too. If necessary, your doctor can test your nasal secretions to confirm you have hay fever, and an allergist can conduct tests to identify which pollens cause the most problems for you.

What you can do

- Stay indoors on dry, windy days or when pollen counts are high. Pollen counts are often reported daily in the media.
- Rid your home of pollen traps, such as carpeting or dirty air filters.
- Try over-the-counter (OTC) antihistamines to relieve mild symptoms. Antihistamines can make you drowsy, so never use them when driving or using heavy machinery. Nasal decongestant sprays will help dry up your runny nose, but they also cause the symptoms to worsen so you should never use them for more than three consecutive days (see *Home Pharmacy*, p. 364).

Final notes

- Hay fever can develop at any age. While irritating, hay fever symptoms will go away when the offending pollen disappears at the end of the season.

know
WHAT
TO DO

Hay fever

DO THESE APPLY:

- Symptoms interfere with daily routine
- Symptoms are not relieved with over-the-counter (OTC) medications
- You have hay fever and develop symptoms of sinusitis
- You have hay fever and develop symptoms of an ear infection

YES ▶

CALL DOCTOR

──── **NO** ────

see *What You Can Do*

see *The Common Cold*, p. 182

see *Sinusitis*, p. 188

see *Middle Ear Infection*, p. 193

see *Home Pharmacy*, p. 364

APPLY SELF-CARE

CHEST/RESPIRATORY

Chest pain

More than a "heartache"

Chest pain is often associated with the heart and can be a frightening symptom. Although this discomfort may be a warning from your heart and must be handled correctly, there are many other causes of chest pain that are less serious and easier to treat. Knowing the different types of chest pain can help you make safer decisions and get faster relief. **All chest pain should be taken seriously.**

HEART PAIN

Sharp pain from the heart may be caused by an infection in the outer lining (*pericarditis*), or inner lining (*endocarditis*). This often follows an infection in another part of the body. *Palpitations* can cause sudden, brief jabs of pain, usually in the left side of the chest (see *Palpitations*, p. 222).

Angina pectoris is a warning that the heart muscle is not getting enough oxygen. Anginal pain is a tightness, squeezing or feeling of pressure over the front of the chest. It may also be felt up in the throat and jaws or down one or both arms. It usually comes on with exertion, stress or overeating and lasts less than 15 minutes. **Any angina means that the heart is in trouble; the pain does not have to be severe to be serious.**

HEART ATTACK

Chest pain that is crushing, squeezing or increasing in pressure may be a warning of heart attack, known as *myocardial infarction*. The pain is like angina, and may not be severe, but it continues for more than 15 minutes and is not eased with rest. It is often accompanied by nausea, sweating, dizziness, shortness of breath and a feeling of doom or danger. The symptoms are caused by a completely blocked coronary artery which stops blood flow to a part of the heart muscle.

CHEST-WALL PAIN

The chest wall includes skin, muscles, ligaments, ribs and rib cartilage. Pain can be caused by infection, inflammation, bruises, strains, sprains and broken ribs. Chest-wall pain is usually sharp or knife-like and limited to a small area. It often comes and goes for days; touching, bending, stretching, coughing or taking a deep breath may cause the pain to start or increase.

NON-HEART PAIN

Anxiety is a common cause of chest pain. It may be a sharp jab or dull pressure and it is often located in the left chest area. Pain from *hyperventilation* (excessive rapid breathing) often causes or comes with anxiety (see *Hyperventilation Syndrome*, p. 351).

Chest pain can be from the lungs, *pleura* (the thin membranes that cover the lungs), esophagus, diaphragm or several of the organs in the upper abdomen. Pain from the lungs and pleura is similar to chest-wall pain and frequently follows a cold or flu-like illness. Lung diseases like pneumonia, blood clots and asthma may produce chest pain.

If the discomfort is caused by the esophagus or the stomach, there may be an acid taste in the mouth and a burning feeling in the chest that improves with eating.

Prevention

There are many causes of chest pain, and prevention is not possible for all of them. However, good health habits decrease your risk of illness and improve your chances of quick, full recovery.

- Maintain normal body weight (see *Eating Right*, p. 373).
- Follow a low-fat, well-balanced diet (see *Eating Right*, p. 373).
- Exercise regularly (see *Staying Active*, p. 372).
- If you smoke, start taking steps to kick the habit (see *Quit Smoking*, p. 375).
- Have regular checkups to help detect any health problems early (see *Screening Guidelines*, p. 378).
- Learn about any chronic illness you have and follow your doctor's advice (see *Becoming Partners With Your Doctor*, p. 385).
- Learn about stress and stress management (see *Stress*, p. 349).

What you can do

- Learn CPR (see *CPR*, p. 20) and know what to do for emergencies (see *Emergencies Introduction*, p. 18).

- Try to identify what may be causing your pain and avoid that activity or food.

- If chest-wall pain is from an injury, treat with **RICE** process (see *Strains And Sprains*, p. 72) and take aspirin or ibuprofen for pain and inflammation. **NEVER give aspirin to children/teenagers. It can cause Reye's syndrome, a rare but often fatal condition.**

- If pain is from stress or hyperventilation, follow stress-reduction methods (see *Stress*, p. 349).

- Pain from stomach or esophagus may be relieved by:
  - Eating smaller meals
  - Stopping smoking
  - Avoiding foods and drugs that seem to trigger pain
  - Raising the head of your bed on four- to six-inch blocks and not eating for at least one hour before bedtime
  - Taking antacids (follow directions on the package)

see *Abdominal/Gastrointestinal*, p. 238

know
WHAT
TO DO

Chest pain
DO THESE APPLY:

- Crushing, squeezing or increasing pressure in chest
- Chest discomfort with:
    - Shortness of breath
    - Dizziness
    - Sweating
    - Nausea or vomiting
    - Pain in jaw, neck, shoulders or arms
    - Rapid or irregular pulse
- Chronic heart disease exists and chest pain is not relieved with nitroglycerin medication

Rest quietly with head elevated on pillows; keep warm.

Wait for emergency transport or as advised by emergency system.

YES

SEEK EMERGENCY CARE

APPLY EMERGENCY FIRST AID

— NO —

- Chest-wall pain with fever
- Chest pain and cough with rust-colored or brown sputum
- Chronic heart disease and chest pain is more frequent, more intense or present during times of rest

YES

CALL DOCTOR NOW

— NO —

- Symptoms worsen or have not improved after 48 hours of self-care

YES

CALL DOCTOR

— NO —

see *What You Can Do*

APPLY SELF-CARE

Palpitations

When your heart skips a beat

Everyone feels a skip, flutter, flip-flop, thump or pounding in their chest at times. These feelings are *palpitations* and are caused by a change in your normal heart rhythm; they can be extra full, very strong, rapid or irregular beats.

Causes of palpitations include hyperventilation, anxiety, fever, excess thyroid, stimulants such as caffeine and nicotine, alcohol and many drugs and medicines. Palpitations, or *arrhythmias*, can occur in some types of heart disease. In most cases, palpitations are brief, harmless and go away without treatment.

Prevention

- Exercise regularly (see *Staying Active*, p. 372).
- If you smoke, start taking steps to kick the habit (see *Quit Smoking*, p. 375).
- Limit the amount of alcohol (see *Alcohol And Drugs*, p. 375) and caffeine you drink.
- Read warnings on packages and labels of all drugs you take.
- Do what you can to control your stress (see *Stress*, p. 349).
- Have regular checkups to help detect and treat health problems early (see *Screening Guidelines*, p. 378).

What you can do

- Look for the cause of your palpitations. Do they come after consuming certain foods or beverages? At a specific time of day? During or following a certain activity? Eliminate the possible cause and see if it takes care of the problem.
- Ask your doctor or pharmacist about side effects of your medications.
- Follow the prevention guidelines listed above.
- Relax and remember that most palpitations are harmless.

Palpitations

DO THESE APPLY:

Positive history of heart or blood vessel disease, or no apparent cause of palpitations and:

- **Shortness of breath**
- **Crushing, squeezing or increasing pressure in chest**
- **Fainting**

While waiting, rest quietly with head elevated on pillows unless faint. If faint, lie flat with feet elevated higher than heart level.

YES →

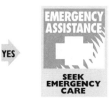

SEEK EMERGENCY CARE

APPLY EMERGENCY FIRST AID

— **NO** —

Positive history of heart or blood vessel disease, or no apparent cause of palpitations and:

- **Fatigue**
- **Weakness or feeling faint**
- **Light-headedness or dizziness**
- **Confusion**
- **A sensation of impending doom**
- **Palpitations increasing in severity or lasting longer**

YES →

CALL DOCTOR NOW

— **NO** —

see next page

4

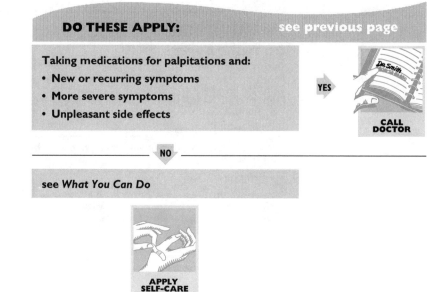

DO THESE APPLY: see previous page

Taking medications for palpitations and:
- New or recurring symptoms
- More severe symptoms
- Unpleasant side effects

YES

CALL DOCTOR

NO

see *What You Can Do*

APPLY SELF-CARE

Hypertension

Also known as "the silent killer"

Hypertension, or high blood pressure, is known as "the silent killer." Although it is very common and can lead to serious health problems — such as heart attack and stroke — it often goes undetected. The best way to detect hypertension is to have your blood pressure checked regularly.

Your blood pressure normally goes up and down, depending on your activities and emotions. A "normal" blood pressure reading depends on several factors, such as age, gender and race. But for most adults, a normal reading is 120/80. The first number refers to *systolic* pressure, when the heart contracts; the second to *diastolic* pressure, when the heart is between beats.

Hypertension is usually defined as consistent readings of 140/90 or higher. Most hypertension is called "primary," which means that the exact cause is unknown. Hypertension may be caused by other conditions — such as diabetes, kidney disease, or side effects of certain medications.

What you can do

DETECTING HYPERTENSION

- Have your blood pressure checked regularly — at least every two years for adults.
- If you are at risk of developing hypertension or heart disease because of high cholesterol, diabetes or family history, have your blood pressure checked once a year. *(Screening clinics and some dental clinics can provide easy access to blood pressure information.)*

LIFESTYLE CHANGES

Studies indicate that many people with slightly elevated blood pressure can bring about significant reductions in hypertension through lifestyle changes:

- Get regular aerobic exercise (see *Staying Active*, p. 372). *Check with your doctor before beginning an exercise program.*
- Lose weight if you are overweight.

- Restrict dietary salt intake to no more than 3,000 mg per day (about one and a half teaspoons) and reduce dietary fats, especially saturated fats (see *Eating Right*, p. 373).
- Eliminate or restrict alcohol consumption to less than two ounces per day (see *Alcohol And Drugs*, p. 375).
- If you smoke, start taking steps to kick the habit (see *Quit Smoking*, p. 375). *Call CareWise for smoking cessation support materials.*

MEDICATIONS

If you are diagnosed with high blood pressure, your doctor may use the "stepped approach" to treatment, beginning with *diuretics* (medication known as water pills that increases fluid loss) and progressing to drugs that act directly on the blood vessels, heart and blood chemistry.

The goal of medical treatment is to control hypertension while creating as few side effects as possible.

Final notes

It's crucial that you comply with the treatment program your doctor prescribes if you are diagnosed with hypertension. If you have problems with any part of the program, discuss them with your doctor. Long-term follow-up care is important. Your doctor will decide how often follow-up visits should be scheduled, based on the severity of your hypertension, treatment response and other factors.

Hypertension

DO THESE APPLY:

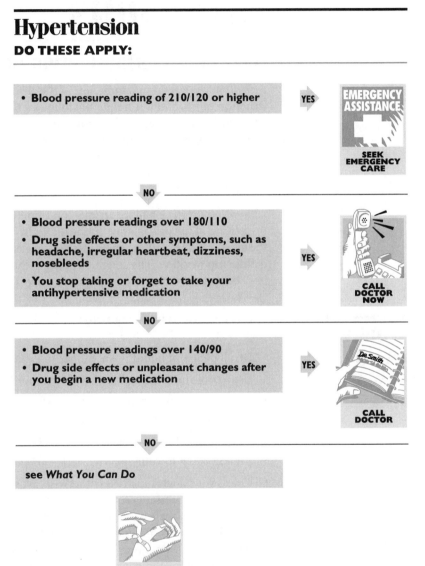

• Blood pressure reading of 210/120 or higher

YES → **SEEK EMERGENCY CARE**

NO

• Blood pressure readings over 180/110
• Drug side effects or other symptoms, such as headache, irregular heartbeat, dizziness, nosebleeds
• You stop taking or forget to take your antihypertensive medication

YES → **CALL DOCTOR NOW**

NO

• Blood pressure readings over 140/90
• Drug side effects or unpleasant changes after you begin a new medication

YES → **CALL DOCTOR**

NO

see *What You Can Do*

APPLY SELF-CARE

Bronchitis

A common inflammation of the lungs

Acute bronchitis is an inflammation of the airways that results from irritation or infection. It frequently follows a bout with the flu or a cold, and may last up to two weeks. Bronchitis is usually characterized by a cough accompanied by soreness and tightness in the chest. The cough is often dry at first, but becomes productive after a few days. The presence of yellow, gray-green or rust-colored sputum (phlegm) may indicate a bacterial infection.

Chronic bronchitis is a more serious condition that involves a permanent thickening of the passageways to the lungs. In both types, the cells lining the inside of the breathing passages that normally sweep away mucus and debris stop working. The cough response is the body's way of ridding itself of these irritants (see *Emphysema, Wheezing,* p. 232).

What you can do

- If you smoke, start taking steps to kick the habit (see *Quit Smoking,* p. 375).
- Drink plenty of liquids — about six to eight glasses per day.
- Use a cool-mist vaporizer to help keep your lungs clear.
- Avoid respiratory irritants. If you must work around them, use a respirator or other protective gear.
- Get plenty of rest to enable your lungs to heal.
- Eat according to your appetite.
- Unless your doctor instructs otherwise, avoid around-the-clock usage of cough suppressants containing dextromethorphan or codeine, or with "DM" in their name. Coughing can actually help eliminate secretions from your airways. An over-the-counter (OTC) cough syrup will only temporarily relieve a cough, it won't cure it. Old-fashioned home remedies (tea with honey) may provide similar relief.
- Don't use medicines containing antihistimines if you will be driving or operating machinery, since these preparations make you drowsy.

see *Home Pharmacy,* p. 364

Bronchitis

DO THESE APPLY:

- **Significant respiratory distress — such as rapid breathing or difficulty breathing and/or bluish discoloration to the skin**

YES → SEEK EMERGENCY CARE

NO

- **You develop symptoms of pneumonia:**
  - **Relapse or second rise of fever**
  - **Chest pain associated with breathing or coughing, or difficulty breathing**
  - **Coughing rust-colored sputum**
  - **Blue-tinged lips or fingertips**
  - **Rapid or labored breathing in child**

  see *Pneumonia*, page 235

YES → CALL DOCTOR NOW

NO

- **Symptoms worsen or don't improve:**
  - **Cough often wakes you**
  - **Sore chest from coughing**
  - **Cough with fever doesn't improve after four or five days**
- **Chest discomfort leaves you short of breath**
- **Chronic heart or lung problems**
- **Yellow, gray-green sputum**
- **Wheezing**
- **Cough lingers for seven to 10 days after other symptoms have cleared**

YES → CALL DOCTOR

NO

see *What You Can Do*

 APPLY SELF-CARE

4

Influenza

A highly contagious virus

Influenza, also known as *flu* or *grippe*, is a highly contagious respiratory disease caused by viral infection. Symptoms are similar to those of a common cold (fever above 101° F, chills, cough, stuffy nose, watery eyes, muscular aches, nausea, sore throat), but more severe. There is no treatment for flu, except to reduce your symptoms while your body fights off the infection.

Flu infection often occurs in epidemics during the "flu season," which generally lasts from late fall to early spring. Flu is spread by inhaling virus-laden droplets when an infected person sneezes, coughs or even talks. You can also get the flu by touching articles contaminated by contact with an infected person. Influenza is most commonly spread in enclosed environments.

Prevention

Getting a "flu shot" reduces the incidence of infection and is particularly important for people at high risk — infants, older adults, people with chronic diseases or impaired immune systems, and women in the last three months of pregnancy. A drug called *amantadine* can sometimes be effective in preventing development of certain strains of flu. If you are in one of the high-risk groups, call your doctor early in the fall to discuss preventive treatment.

What you can do

- Take aspirin, acetaminophen (Tylenol) or ibuprofen to relieve aches and pains. **NEVER give aspirin to children/teenagers. It can cause Reye's syndrome, a rare but often fatal condition.**
- Drink plenty of clear liquids — water, juice, ginger ale — to restore fluids.
- Drink chicken soup, bouillon and other salty liquids to help combat dizziness and restore fluids.
- Gargle with warm salt water (one-half teaspoon of salt added to eight ounces of water), drink tea with honey or lemon, or use lozenges to soothe sore throat pain.
- Get plenty of rest.
- Antihistamines or decongestants may help relieve runny nose and watery eyes.

know
WHAT
TO DO

Influenza
DO THESE APPLY:

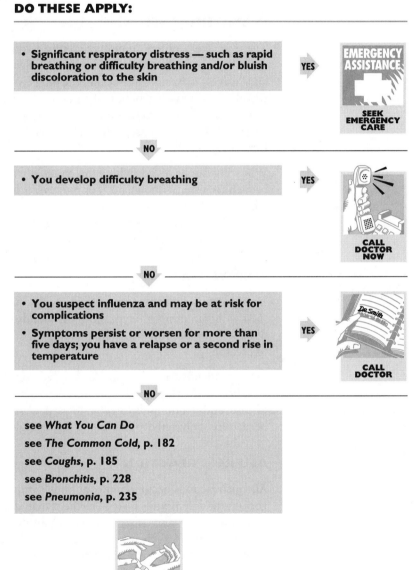

• **Significant respiratory distress — such as rapid breathing or difficulty breathing and/or bluish discoloration to the skin**   YES

EMERGENCY ASSISTANCE

SEEK EMERGENCY CARE

NO

• **You develop difficulty breathing**   YES

CALL DOCTOR NOW

NO

• **You suspect influenza and may be at risk for complications**
• **Symptoms persist or worsen for more than five days; you have a relapse or a second rise in temperature**   YES

CALL DOCTOR

NO

see *What You Can Do*

see *The Common Cold*, p. 182

see *Coughs*, p. 185

see *Bronchitis*, p. 228

see *Pneumonia*, p. 235

APPLY SELF-CARE

Wheezing

A warning whistle

The respiratory system resembles an upside-down tree with the "trunk" at the throat and the "limbs" (*bronchi*), smaller "branches" (*bronchioles*), and "leaves" (*alveoli* or air sacs) in the lungs. Wheezing is a high-pitched whistle caused by obstruction of air as it moves through the bronchi and bronchioles. The restriction may be due to narrowing of the airway walls or a blockage in the passage. It can be localized in a small area or spread throughout the lungs.

Wheezing can be heard in lung infections such as pneumonia or bronchitis, when a foreign body or mucus blocks an airway, and in people who have asthma. It is also a symptom of allergic reactions or chronic lung disease. Wheezing can be a warning of a very serious problem and needs professional evaluation when it first occurs.

EMPHYSEMA

Emphysema is a chronic obstructive lung disease in which the alveoli lose their ability to transfer oxygen into the bloodstream and remove carbon dioxide. They become enlarged, trapping air and decreasing the capacity to breathe.

Most frequently caused by smoking, emphysema results from chronic irritation to the respiratory system. There is no cure for this progressive disease, and treatment is directed toward decreasing the amount of air needed for daily activity and easing the struggle to breathe.

ALLERGIC REACTION

Allergic reactions occur when your body's immune system reacts and goes on the defensive against an element that, under most circumstances, is harmless. Allergens trigger your body's antibodies to counterattack and release chemicals, such as *histamine*, directly into various body tissues. Your symptoms are the result of tissues reacting to these chemicals.

Wheezing can be created by spasms in bronchial and bronchiolar walls, swelling in the wall lining and production of excess mucus. *This can be a serious allergic reaction which can quickly become life-threatening.*

Wheezing is the prominent symptom in asthma, a serious allergic disorder (see *Asthma,* p. 213). Wheezing brought on by an allergic reaction can be an emergency situation.

Prevention

- If you smoke, start taking steps to kick the habit (see *Quit Smoking,* p. 375).
- Avoid respiratory irritants such as secondary smoke or chronic exposure to fumes.
- Avoid anything that has triggered an allergic attack in the past (see *Allergies,* p. 210).
- Wear or carry medical-alert identification related to your allergies and any chronic disease.
- Inform all doctors, dentists and pharmacists of your allergies.
- Ask your doctor about pneumonia and flu vaccinations (see *Immunization Schedule,* p. 377).
- Exercise regularly (see *Staying Active,* p. 372). Swimming and water aerobics are especially good for building up your respiratory strength.
- Learn stress-management techniques if stress is a factor in your wheezing (see *Stress,* p. 349).
- Maintain normal weight to avoid additional stress on your respiratory system.
- Contact your doctor or a CareWise Nurse for information about prevention and treatment of your specific wheezing problem.

What you can do

- Drink at least two quarts of water daily to thin bronchial mucus.
- Maintain a humid environment with a cool-mist vaporizer.
- Learn and use relaxation techniques (see *Stress,* p. 349). Anxiety and panic increase breathing distress and waste energy.
- Use your peak-flow meter, bronchodilators and other medications as directed by your doctor. Do not wait for early symptoms to go away on their own.

Wheezing

DO THESE APPLY:

- Signs of a severe allergic reaction:
    - **Wheezing or difficulty breathing**
    - **Swelling around mouth, eyes, throat, tongue or excess swelling near insect sting**
    - **Severe rash or hives; skin reddened or itching**
    - **Extreme difficulty breathing**

YES → **SEEK EMERGENCY CARE**

NO

- **First episode of acute wheezing**
- **Wheezing is more severe or not responding to usual treatment**
- **Chest pain with coughing or difficulty breathing**
- **Sputum becomes yellow, gray-green or rust-colored**
- **Blue-tinged lips or fingertips**
- **Fever of 100° F with wheezing**
- **Other chronic health problem such as heart disease present**
- **Wheezing soon after dose of new medication (Do not take another dose of medicine.)**

YES → **CALL DOCTOR NOW**

NO

- **Wheezing requires more medication and treatment to control or prevent**
- **More information and education needed to understand and control wheezing**

YES → **CALL DOCTOR**

NO

see *What You Can Do*; see *Hives*, p. 139; see *Asthma*, p. 213; see *Hay Fever*, p. 216; see *Chest-Wall Pain*, p. 219; see *Bronchitis*, p. 228; see *Pneumonia*, p. 235

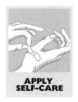

APPLY SELF-CARE

Pneumonia

Infections of the lung

Pneumonia is a general term that refers to more than 50 types of lung diseases caused either by viral or bacterial infection. About two million people in the United States get pneumonia each year, and 40,000 to 70,000 die from it annually. Bacteria-caused pneumonia can be effectively treated with antibiotics, but virus-caused pneumonia isn't helped by such treatment.

Note your symptoms

Most forms of pneumonia are characterized by:

- Chills
- Fever of 100.5° F or greater
- Chest pain associated with coughing or breathing
- Coughing
- Bone and joint pain
- Rattling sounds in lungs (*rales*)
- Blue-tinged skin

Other symptoms that may be present are:

- Loss of appetite
- Headache
- Yellow, gray-green or rust-colored sputum (phlegm)

Prevention

A vaccine is available to protect against the leading cause of bacterial pneumonia in adults, and it is recommended for everyone older than 65, those without a spleen or anyone with a chronic disease. Contact your doctor or local public health department (see *Immunization Schedule*, p. 377).

What you can do

- Take aspirin, acetaminophen (Tylenol) or ibuprofen. **NEVER give aspirin to children/teenagers. It can cause Reye's syndrome, a rare but often fatal condition.**

- Drink plenty of clear liquids.

- Drink chicken soup, bouillon and other salty liquids to restore fluids and minimize dizziness when you stand.

- Use a cool-mist vaporizer.

- Get plenty of rest.

- Eat according to your appetite.

- Check with your doctor to see if there is a risk of infecting others. Stay home if advised to do so.

Pneumonia

DO THESE APPLY:

• **Significant respiratory distress — such as rapid breathing or difficulty breathing and/or bluish discoloration to the skin**

YES → **EMERGENCY ASSISTANCE**

SEEK EMERGENCY CARE

— **NO** —

• **Rapid or labored breathing**

• **Bluish tinge to your skin**

• **Chest pain associated with coughing or breathing**

• **Cough that produces yellow, gray-green or rust-colored sputum (phlegm)**

YES →

CALL DOCTOR NOW

— **NO** —

• **Symptoms worsen or persist for five days or more**

• **Fever or chills**

• **Loss of appetite**

• **Rattling sound in the lungs**

• **Bone and joint pain**

YES →

CALL DOCTOR

— **NO** —

see *What You Can Do*

APPLY SELF-CARE

ABDOMINAL/ GASTROINTESTINAL

Heartburn

A very common burning sensation

Heartburn is caused by the flow of gastric acid from the stomach into the *esophagus*, the food pipe that runs from the throat into the stomach. The pain associated with heartburn (a burning sensation) typically spreads from the upper abdomen into the lower breastbone, and occurs most often after meals or when lying down. Sometimes, sour or bitter material is regurgitated into the mouth.

About 10% of adults experience heartburn weekly and about 30% experience it monthly. Pregnant women are particularly susceptible because of hormonal changes in pregnancy and increased pressure on the abdomen caused by the fetus.

What you can do

Observe your symptoms and determine whether you have heartburn by ruling out other, more serious sources of pain. If you don't suspect a more serious problem, begin self-care:

- Avoid irritants such as coffee, tea, alcohol, aspirin and ibuprofen.

- Avoid foods containing acid, such as citrus fruits and tomatoes.

- If you smoke, start taking steps to kick the habit. (Call CareWise for smoking cessation support materials.)

- Do what you can to reduce your stress level, and try to make meals a time of relaxation (see *Stress*, p. 349).

- Sit — don't stand or lie down — while eating.
- Don't lie down right after eating. If nighttime heartburn is a problem, don't eat anything for at least two hours before going to bed. Elevate the head of the bed with four- to six-inch blocks to incline your body and prevent acid from flowing from the stomach and into the esophagus.
- Don't wear tight-fitting clothing, such as tight jeans or girdles.
- Antacids such as Maalox, Mylanta, Gelusil or Tums can often provide fast, temporary relief. (**If you have high blood pressure or heart disease, don't use antacids with sodium salts without consulting your doctor.**)

Final notes

Some people who are prone to heartburn may suffer repeated attacks. Chronic severe symptoms may lead to complications, including a pre-cancerous condition. However, with self-care you can easily treat the symptoms of simple heartburn with no lasting ill effects.

see *Know What To Do*, p. 240

Heartburn

DO THESE APPLY:

• **Crushing, squeezing or increasing pressure in chest** see *Chest Pain*, p. 218 • **Deep red (maroon), black or tar-like stools**	**YES** → **SEEK EMERGENCY CARE**

NO

• **Severe heartburn pain** • **Pain seems to extend through your back** • **Painful or difficult swallowing**	**YES** → **CALL DOCTOR NOW**

NO

• **Heartburn pain not relieved by self-care** • **Heartburn pain lasts more than three days** • **Heartburn pain recurs frequently** • **You suspect a prescribed medication causes your heartburn**	**YES** → **CALL DOCTOR**

NO

see *What You Can Do*

APPLY SELF-CARE

Nausea and vomiting

Can have serious side effects

Nausea is most often traced to a viral infection or "stomach flu" that produces a queasy stomach, increased salivation and sweating. When the nausea intensifies, you may begin to vomit. The condition can also be the result of medications, stress, pregnancy, food poisoning or a head injury. Because nausea and vomiting can be connected with so many medical problems — some of them serious — it's important to watch your symptoms closely.

Note your symptoms

The most dangerous threat posed by vomiting is dehydration (see *Dehydration,* p. 262), which can occur quickly, particularly in infants, young children and older adults. Severe dehydration can be life-threatening and symptoms should be carefully monitored.

Signs of dehydration include:

- Unusual thirst
- Sunken-looking eyes
- Dry mouth and cracked lips
- Infrequent urination or dark yellow urine
- Skin that is no longer elastic

Also suspect more serious medical conditions if:

- Vomiting bright red blood or what looks like coffee grounds (see *Peptic Ulcer,* p. 249)
- Abdominal pain is severe or pain is localized in one area (see *Abdominal Pain,* p. 264)
- Vomiting is accompanied by headache and stiff neck (see *Meningitis,* p. 271)

Some nausea and vomiting can be traced to food poisoning, which is often confused with viral stomach flu (see *Stomach Flu And Food Poisoning*, p. 244). Certain foods, when not stored or handled properly, are breeding grounds for bacteria that can inflame the intestines.

Suspect food poisoning if:

- Your symptoms are shared by others who ate the same food
- Nausea and vomiting begin six to 48 hours after eating food that may not have been stored correctly

What you can do

GIVE YOUR STOMACH A BREAK

- Don't eat for four hours after vomiting.
- For the next 12 to 24 hours, slowly sip clear liquids, such as flat ginger ale, or suck on ice chips.
- Watch for signs of dehydration, especially in older adults.
- Slowly reintroduce soup, Jell-O, dry toast, applesauce and other bland foods.
- Get plenty of rest.
- Infants and children are prime candidates for dehydration. Offer bottles of water or diluted juice to infants, but don't encourage your baby to drink large amounts at one time. Try Popsicles or frozen fruit bars for children once you start reintroducing food.

Final notes

While patience and self-care normally do the trick for an upset stomach, it's important to be alert for serious and sudden complications.

Nausea and vomiting

DO THESE APPLY:

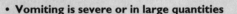

- **Vomiting bright red blood or what looks like coffee grounds**

  see *Peptic Ulcer,* p. 249

- **Headache and stiff neck**

  see *Meningitis,* p. 271

YES

EMERGENCY ASSISTANCE

SEEK EMERGENCY CARE

NO

- **Vomiting is severe or in large quantities**
- **Severe abdominal pain**

  see *Abdominal Pain,* p. 264

- **Signs of dehydration**

  see *Dehydration,* p. 262

- **Nausea and vomiting occur for more than two hours after head injury**

  see *Head/Spinal Injury,* p. 60

YES

CALL DOCTOR NOW

NO

- **Medication may be to blame**
- **Pregnancy possible**

YES

CALL DOCTOR

NO

see *What You Can Do*

APPLY SELF-CARE

Stomach flu and food poisoning

Symptoms are similar

Stomach flu and food poisoning have different causes but many of the same symptoms. However, they both fall under the general category of *gastroenteritis*, which is commonly caused by food-borne bacteria, or by viruses spread — hand-to-mouth — by contaminated objects.

Symptoms — vomiting, diarrhea, abdominal cramping and fever — usually take three to 36 hours to develop, with the resulting illness lasting 12 hours to several days.

For poisoning not related to food, see *Poisoning*, p. 28.

Prevention

STOMACH FLU

- Maximize your resistance to infection with a healthy diet, plenty of rest and regular exercise.
- Wash your hands frequently.
- Keep your hands away from your nose, eyes and mouth.

FOOD POISONING

- Carefully refrigerate (between 34° F and 40° F) all foods — especially poultry, fish, meats, eggs and salads made with mayonnaise. Don't eat anything that has been kept between 40° F and 140° F for more than two hours.
- Defrost foods in the microwave or refrigerator — not on the kitchen counter.
- Avoid foods made with raw eggs, as well as rare or uncooked meats.
- Be especially careful with large, cooked meats like the holiday turkey. Refrigerate leftovers as soon as dinner is over. Remove thick bones and cut meat into portions less than three inches thick to speed cooling.

- Thoroughly reheat leftover meats before re-serving to destroy any bacteria.
- All utensils that have touched raw meat should be washed in hot, soapy water before reusing. Wash hands, counter tops and cutting boards frequently.
- Follow home-canning and freezing instructions carefully. Throw out any cans or jars that have leaks or bulging lids.

What you can do

- Do not eat solid foods while vomiting persists.
- For diarrhea, recent studies indicate that introducing solid foods early — after 24 hours — can help control symptoms. Try the BRAT diet (see *Diarrhea*, p. 258).
- Drink plenty of clear liquids in small sips.
- Do not take aspirin or other pain relievers.
- If you suspect food poisoning, check with anyone else who may have eaten the same food. When possible, save a sample of the suspected food in case analysis becomes necessary.

For additional self-care, see *Nausea And Vomiting* (p. 241); *Diarrhea* (p. 258); *Dehydration* (p. 262).

> Many forms of bacteria can cause food poisoning, including *salmonella* (typically found in dairy products, eggs, poultry, red meat and seafood) and *E. coli* (most commonly found in improperly cooked ground meats). A rare but fatal form of food poisoning called *botulism* is usually caused by eating foods with a low-acidity content — such as corn and beans — that have been improperly home-canned.

see *Know What To Do*, p. 246

4

know
**WHAT
TO DO**

Stomach flu and food poisoning

DO THESE APPLY:

- Suspect food poisoning from a canned food (blurred or double vision, or difficulty swallowing or breathing)
- Signs of dehydration

  see *Dehydration*, p. 262
- Severe vomiting or diarrhea that is bloody

YES →

EMERGENCY ASSISTANCE

SEEK EMERGENCY CARE

---- **NO** ----

- Vomiting or diarrhea that lasts longer than one to two days and is not improving
- Vomiting or diarrhea in an infant or child, with signs of dehydration: tearless and sunken eyes, sticky saliva, dry skin, decreased urine output, abnormal drowsiness

YES →

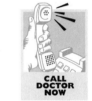

CALL DOCTOR NOW

---- **NO** ----

see *What You Can Do*

APPLY SELF-CARE

Gastritis

Minor lifestyle changes can soothe this stomachache

Gastritis is a painful inflammation of the lining of the stomach. This may occur more frequently with advancing age.

Causes include acute stress, alcohol abuse, viral or bacterial infections, or nonsteroidal anti-inflammatory drugs (NSAIDs), such as aspirin or ibuprofen.

Symptoms may include upper abdominal pain, diarrhea, nausea and vomiting bright red blood or what looks like coffee grounds.

What you can do

- Take over-the-counter (OTC) antacids to provide possible relief from the pain.
- Moderate your use of tobacco, alcohol and caffeinated drinks (see *Getting And Staying Healthy*, p. 372).
- Avoid foods that may trigger gastritis, such as pickles or spices (the type of food can vary from person to person).
- Avoid NSAIDs and other drugs that cause or worsen gastritis (see *Home Pharmacy*, p. 364).

Final notes

If over-the-counter (OTC) medications do not relieve the pain, your doctor may recommend a more powerful prescription drug.

Gastritis is generally not serious. In most cases, the pain will stop spontaneously or after minor lifestyle changes.

see *Know What To Do*, p. 248

Gastritis
DO THESE APPLY:

- **Crushing, squeezing or increasing pressure in chest**

  see *Chest Pain*, p. 218

- **Vomiting bright red blood or what looks like coffee grounds**

YES ➤ **EMERGENCY ASSISTANCE**

SEEK EMERGENCY CARE

--- **NO** ---

- **You have persistent or moderate to severe symptoms of gastritis, such as upper abdominal pain, diarrhea, nausea and vomiting**

YES ➤ **CALL DOCTOR NOW**

--- **NO** ---

- **Symptoms of gastritis persist or worsen despite use of over-the-counter (OTC) antacids and other self-care**

YES ➤ **CALL DOCTOR**

--- **NO** ---

see *What You Can Do*

APPLY SELF-CARE

Peptic ulcer

An often-painful condition

Peptic ulcers are craters or eroded areas in the protective lining of the stomach or intestine that are caused by excess stomach acids and other irritants. The most common type of peptic ulcer is called a *duodenal ulcer*, appearing in the upper part of the small intestine. Severe ulcers can lead to pain, bleeding and even perforations — holes — in the wall of the stomach or intestine. **A perforated ulcer is life-threatening and must be surgically treated immediately**.

Ulcers have been associated with bacterial infections, cigarette smoking and the use of certain drugs. Aspirin, ibuprofen and corticosteroids are known to cause ulcers in some people.

With the significant advances in treatment and with early detection, most people will recover from their ulcer in four to six weeks.

Antacids in a dosage recommended by your doctor may efficiently treat your ulcer.

What you can do

To reduce the likelihood of getting an ulcer and speed the healing process if you already have one:

- If you smoke, start taking steps to kick the habit, and avoid coffee, alcohol, aspirin and ibuprofen.

- Avoid hot or spicy foods if they cause discomfort; for the most part you can eat a normal diet.

- Don't drink large amounts of milk. Calcium may stimulate acid production.

- For temporary relief from ulcer pain, try over-the-counter (OTC) antacids such as Maalox or Mylanta.

Tell your doctor if you have a history of ulcers. Common medications taken for other ailments could increase your risk of ulcer recurrences.

see *Know What To Do*, p. 250

Peptic ulcer

DO THESE APPLY:

- Crushing, squeezing or increasing pressure in chest

  see *Chest Pain*, p. 218

- Vomiting bright red blood or what looks like coffee grounds

- Cold, clammy skin with fainting

  see *Shock*, p. 42

- Deep red (maroon), black or tar-like stools

YES ▶ **EMERGENCY ASSISTANCE**

SEEK EMERGENCY CARE

--- **NO** ---

- Severe pain, nausea and vomiting

YES ▶

CALL DOCTOR NOW

--- **NO** ---

- Burning, aching pain in lower chest, upper abdomen (often relieved by food or antacids)

- Nausea and vomiting

- Feeling excessive fullness after meals

- Chronic anxiety or stress seems to worsen recurrence of previously treated ulcer

YES ▶

CALL DOCTOR

--- **NO** ---

see *What You Can Do*

APPLY SELF-CARE

Hiatal hernia

Self-care is often effective

Hiatal hernia or abdominal hernia is when part of the stomach protrudes above the *diaphragm*, the muscle wall that separates the chest cavity from the abdominal cavity.

Obesity, pregnancy, a low-fiber diet and wearing tight clothes may contribute to this condition.

Most people with a hiatal hernia don't have symptoms, while others experience a burning pain caused by stomach acid entering the esophagus. This tends to be more noticeable while reclining. (You'll want to check for a milk intolerance, which has similar symptoms to a hiatal hernia.)

What you can do

Self-care is often effective in relieving the *reflux* (or flowing back) of acidic stomach contents into the esophagus. Elevate your head while sleeping by using extra pillows or putting four- to six-inch blocks under the upper bed legs. Avoid tight-fitting clothing, reclining after eating, and eating or drinking two hours or less before bedtime.

Most cases of abdominal hernia don't require treatment other than antacids or other medications to relieve heartburn. **Strangulation of the hernia, when part of the stomach gets pinched off, is a dangerous situation that needs immediate surgical repair.**

see *Know What To Do*, p. 252

know
WHAT
TO DO

Hiatal hernia

DO THESE APPLY:

- **Vomiting bright red blood or what looks like coffee grounds**
- **Cold, clammy skin and fainting**

  see *Shock*, p. 42
- **Crushing, squeezing or increasing pressure in chest**

  see *Chest Pain*, p. 218
- **Diagnosed hernia with weakness, pallor, chest pain, or dizziness**

YES

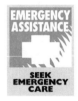

SEEK EMERGENCY CARE

NO

- **Recurring reflux of stomach contents with discomfort that worsens or persists, even after three days of self-care**

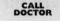
YES

CALL DOCTOR

NO

see *What You Can Do*

see *Heartburn*, p. 238

see *Peptic Ulcer*, p. 249

APPLY SELF-CARE

Inguinal hernia

Prevention and repair

An *inguinal hernia* is when a section of the small intestine protrudes, causing a lump in the groin. In men, the hernia often protrudes into the *scrotum*, the sac that holds the testes. An inguinal hernia usually results from weak abdominal muscles and increased pressure in the abdomen. The combination forces a loop of intestine out through the weak area in the muscle wall. Obesity, heavy lifting and prolonged coughing can bring on a hernia or make it worse.

Symptoms can include swelling in the groin that goes away when lying down or when gentle pressure is applied, and groin pain when bending or lifting.

Strangulation of the hernia, which is when part of the intestine gets pinched off, is an emergency and needs immediate surgical repair.

What you can do

Surgery is the only cure for this type of hernia. Until the hernia is repaired, avoid heavy lifting.

see *Know What To Do*, p. 254

Inguinal hernia
DO THESE APPLY:

- **Diagnosed hernia with increased or severe groin pain, especially if:**
  - **Accompanied by nausea and vomiting**
  - **Hernia feels very tender, won't reduce if pressure applied**

YES → **EMERGENCY ASSISTANCE**
SEEK EMERGENCY CARE

NO ↓

- **Unable to push hernia back into abdominal wall by applying pressure**

YES →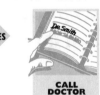
CALL DOCTOR NOW

NO ↓

- **Increasing pain in abdomen, scrotum or groin**
- **Mild groin pain or unexplained groin bump or swelling continues for more than one week**

YES → **CALL DOCTOR**

NO ↓

see *What You Can Do*

APPLY SELF-CARE

Constipation

Can be short-term or chronic

Constipation is a decreased frequency of bowel movements with hard, dry stools. However, there is no set standard for what is normal. Normal for you may be a bowel movement every day or once every three days.

Other symptoms of constipation include difficulty passing stools, abdominal pain and fullness, bloating and gas.

Changes in stools (color, consistency, texture and bulk) are generally not serious. Chronic problems tend to occur more in older adults, who may have inadequate diet and fluid intake.

What you can do

Constipation often can be successfully treated through self-care:

- If your eating habits have changed (other than for medical reasons), go back to the diet you had before the problems began.
- Improve your diet by adding more high-fiber foods, such as whole grains, bran, beans, leafy and raw vegetables, and fruits — especially dried fruits. A high-fiber diet has the added benefit of reducing your blood-cholesterol level and possibly reducing your risk of colon cancer.
- Drink plenty of fluids, especially water.
- Increase your daily exercise, especially if you sit all day at work.
- Investigate ANY medications you are taking to see if they cause constipation (DO NOT stop taking a prescribed medication without consulting your doctor).

If these steps don't work, consider over-the-counter (OTC) remedies such as bulk laxatives that draw water into the stool; milk of magnesia (**not for individuals with kidney problems**); or stool softeners.

Do not give a laxative to a child without checking with your pediatrician.

A reduction in the frequency of bowel movements with no other symptoms does not necessarily require treatment.

see *Know What To Do*, p. 256

Constipation

DO THESE APPLY:

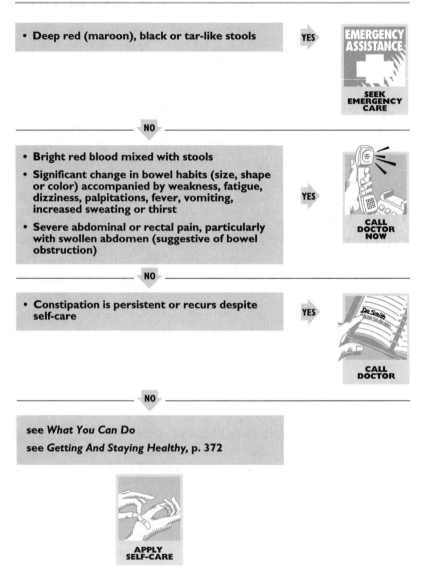

- Deep red (maroon), black or tar-like stools

YES → EMERGENCY ASSISTANCE — SEEK EMERGENCY CARE

NO

- Bright red blood mixed with stools
- Significant change in bowel habits (size, shape or color) accompanied by weakness, fatigue, dizziness, palpitations, fever, vomiting, increased sweating or thirst
- Severe abdominal or rectal pain, particularly with swollen abdomen (suggestive of bowel obstruction)

YES → CALL DOCTOR NOW

NO

- Constipation is persistent or recurs despite self-care

YES → CALL DOCTOR

NO

see *What You Can Do*
see *Getting And Staying Healthy*, p. 372

APPLY SELF-CARE

Hemorrhoids

Self-care is key to initial treatment

Hemorrhoids are swollen, inflamed veins that can be around the outside or the inside of the *anus*. They are extremely common and can be caused or aggravated by constipation, straining to move bowels, obesity, pregnancy or a sedentary lifestyle.

Symptoms may include pain, itching, burning, swelling, bleeding and a sense of incomplete emptying in the rectum. Frequently, hemorrhoidal bleeding is seen as bright red blood on the toilet paper or in the toilet bowl after moving the bowels.

What you can do

Simple self-care is usually the key to initial treatment:

- Keep the anal area clean with pre-moistened towels or "baby wipes."
- *Sitz baths* (soaking in hip-high water) can be soothing.
- Avoid sitting for long periods of time, if possible, or sit on a rubber doughnut. Stretch frequently.
- Over-the-counter (OTC) hydrocortisone creams can reduce swelling and inflammation. Avoid creams with topical anesthetics, since they may slow healing.
- Take steps to avoid constipation and straining to move bowels. Eat high-fiber foods or take over-the-counter (OTC) fiber supplements. Drink plenty of fluids and exercise regularly (see *Getting And Staying Healthy*, p. 372). The occasional use of a mild laxative might be of value, but a better choice is a simple stool softener. Ask your doctor if any medications you are taking could be causing constipation (iron is notorious for this), and if you can take a stool softener to decrease this side effect.

When to call your doctor

See your doctor if you pass significant volumes of deep red (maroon), black or tar-like stools. This could be a sign of more serious gastrointestinal bleeding. If you have any rectal pain, itching or bleeding and have a personal history of ulcers, colonic polyps, or a family history of colon cancer, contact your doctor (see *Peptic Ulcer*, p. 249).

Also, if hemorrhoids don't respond to self-care or you have severe pain and swelling, discuss this with your doctor.

Diarrhea

Dehydration is the greatest risk

Diarrhea (frequent, watery stools) takes place when solid waste is pushed through the intestines before the water in the waste has time to be reabsorbed by the body. Excessive loss of water, called *dehydration* (see *Dehydration*, p. 262), is the biggest health risk to having diarrhea.

Diarrhea is most commonly caused by viral infections. Other causes include bacterial infections and irritations in the digestive tract. It is frequently accompanied by nausea and vomiting (see *Nausea And Vomiting*, p. 241).

Many medications may cause diarrhea, including antibiotics, blood pressure drugs, digitalis, anti-cancer drugs, gold compounds and nonsteroidal anti-inflammatory drugs (NSAIDs) (see *Home Pharmacy*, p. 364; *Using Medications*, p. 362).

DIARRHEA IN CHILDREN

Because of their developing digestive tracts, infants and young children usually experience diarrhea more often than adults. Frequently, runny stools are caused by drinking too much juice or milk or eating too much fruit. If a child seems healthy in every other way, food-intolerance diarrhea is usually not serious and no treatment is required. However, if the diarrhea continues, the food or drink that is causing the diarrhea should be eliminated from the child's diet. Continuing diarrhea also may be a sign of flu or some other ailment (see *Stomach Flu And Food Poisoning*, p. 244).

Because of their small size, children face greater risk of dehydration than adults. Saliva that is dry and sticky may be an early sign of dehydration. A baby whose diaper has not been wet for several hours also could be suffering from dehydration (see *Dehydration*, p. 262).

What you can do

INFANTS AND TODDLERS

- For an infant under 6 months old, discuss any diarrhea with your doctor.

- To avoid dehydration from persistent diarrhea, see that your infant or child drinks twice as much fluid as usual.

- If your infant is bottle-fed, continue to give the usual mealtime feeding and offer a commercially prepared electrolyte drink or *oral rehydrating solution* (ORS) between feedings. Some popular brands are Pedialyte, Rehydralyte and Infalyte. Check to see which your pediatrician prefers.

- If your infant is breast-fed, nurse more frequently and give ORS between feedings.

- Initially offer small amounts (one teaspoon or five milliliters/mls) of ORS in a syringe every five minutes. A child with mild vomiting usually can keep down ORS when given in this manner.

- Avoid juices or sodas since these can actually worsen diarrhea, cause an imbalance of salt in the blood, and put your child at greater risk of dehydration.

- If toddlers are uninterested in drinking, make it a fun activity by offering small amounts in special cups, using colorful straws, letting them spoon it for themselves, using a timer they can set, etc.

- If your toddler is eating table food, the following are especially good for toddlers with diarrhea: unbuttered rice; potatoes or noodles; crackers or toast (depending on age); unsweetened hot or cold cereals; soups with rice or rice, meat and/or vegetables; bananas and applesauce.

- **Do not give Pepto-Bismol, Kaopectate or other anti-diarrhea medications to infants or young children without consulting your doctor.**

ADULTS AND OLDER CHILDREN

- Slowly sip one of the commercially available electrolyte drinks or *oral rehydrating solutions* (ORS) such as Pedialyte, Rehydralyte, etc.

- Avoid juices and sodas since these can actually worsen diarrhea, cause an imbalance of salt in the blood, and increase the risk of dehydration.

- Starches, cereals, yogurt and fresh fruits are OK for older children.

- A common recommendation for adults continues to be to rest the stomach by avoiding solid foods for 24 hours.

- After 24 hours, eat the BRAT diet of constipating foods several times a day in small portions:

    - **B**ananas

    - **R**ice (and rice milk)

    - **A**pplesauce

    - **T**oast

- Avoid spicy foods, alcohol and foods high in fat for several days.

- Adults may take over-the-counter (OTC) preparations like Pepto-Bismol and Kaopectate that will make the stools more solid. However, these medications should be avoided for about the first six hours (since diarrhea sometimes helps speed recovery from certain ailments).

know
WHAT TO DO

Diarrhea
DO THESE APPLY:

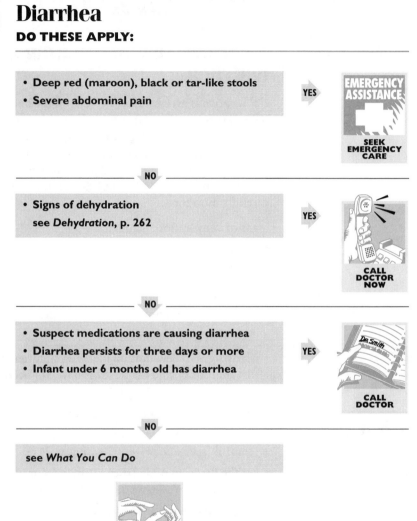

- **Deep red (maroon), black or tar-like stools**
- **Severe abdominal pain**

YES → **EMERGENCY ASSISTANCE**

SEEK EMERGENCY CARE

— NO —

- **Signs of dehydration**
  see *Dehydration*, p. 262

YES → **CALL DOCTOR NOW**

— NO —

- **Suspect medications are causing diarrhea**
- **Diarrhea persists for three days or more**
- **Infant under 6 months old has diarrhea**

YES → **CALL DOCTOR**

— NO —

see *What You Can Do*

APPLY SELF-CARE

Dehydration

A serious risk of vomiting and diarrhea

Dehydration is excessive loss of water in the body and is a dangerous risk of both vomiting (see *Nausea And Vomiting*, p. 241) and diarrhea (see *Diarrhea*, p. 258). It can occur quickly, particularly in infants, young children and older adults. Dehydration also depletes the body of two essential minerals, sodium and potassium, which are *electrolytes*. Severe dehydration can be life-threatening, and symptoms should be carefully monitored.

Signs of dehydration include:

- Unusual thirst

- Sunken-looking eyes

- Dry mouth and cracked lips

- Infrequent urination or dark yellow urine

- Skin that is no longer elastic

- Early signs of dehydration in young children may include saliva that is dry and sticky, and diapers that have not been wet for several hours.

What you can do

To prevent dehydration from occurring or getting worse:

- Drink clear liquids like water and bouillon after vomiting is under control (see *Nausea And Vomiting*, p. 241).

- At the first sign of diarrhea, increase your fluid intake to eight to 10 large glasses of water a day until the diarrhea ends.

- Adults may drink a rehydration fluid like Rehydrolyte to replace lost electrolytes (because of the sodium content, consult your doctor first if you have high blood pressure, heart disease, diabetes, glaucoma or a history of stroke).

- To replace electrolytes in children, try Pedialyte or one of the other children's rehydration fluids, now available in fruit flavors.

- For children who have been vomiting, start with one teaspoon of liquid every 10 minutes for one or two hours, then increase the amount.

know
WHAT
TO DO

Dehydration
DO THESE APPLY:

- **Suspect dehydration in an infant, young child or a person over 60 years of age**
- **Signs of dehydration:**
    - **Unusual thirst**
    - **Sunken-looking eyes**
    - **Dry mouth and cracked lips**
    - **Infrequent urination or dark yellow urine**
    - **Skin that is no longer elastic**

YES ➤
CALL
DOCTOR
NOW

NO

see *What You Can Do*

see *Nausea And Vomiting*, p. 241

see *Diarrhea*, p. 258

APPLY
SELF-CARE

ABDOMINAL PAIN

Abdominal pain can be caused by very minor or very serious conditions, and finding out what is causing the pain can be difficult.

Location of the pain can help determine the cause:

- *Appendix*, pain usually occurs in the lower right abdomen
- *Gallbladder*, pain usually occurs in the upper right abdomen
- *Kidney*, pain usually occurs in the back

However, it's important to remember that there are exceptions.

Appendicitis

A medical emergency

Appendicitis, the most common abdominal emergency, most frequently strikes males between the age of 15 and 25. Accurate diagnosis and rapid treatment can greatly reduce the likelihood of complications and death, usually caused by a burst appendix.

Symptoms usually occur in this order:

- Vague discomfort around and just above the navel; later, a sharper pain in the lower right quarter of the abdomen
- Possible nausea, vomiting, loss of appetite
- Tenderness in the lower right abdomen
- Fever from 99° F to 101° F
- Constipation and, less commonly, diarrhea

Once appendicitis is confirmed, the appendix will probably be removed. This surgery, called an *appendectomy*, is relatively low-risk.

What you can do

If you suspect appendicitis, seek immediate medical attention. Do not use laxatives or apply heat to the area. Both can cause the appendix to rupture more quickly.

see *Know What To Do*, p. 267

Gallbladder disease

You may not even know you have it

The gallbladder stores bile that is made in the liver, then passes the bile on to the intestines to help digest fats. With a high amount of fat and cholesterol in the system, some of the bile may turn into stones. As the bile flows from the gallbladder to the intestines through the bile ducts, these *gallstones* can block the ducts, causing severe pain, local inflammation or *jaundice* (yellow skin). If the stones stay in the gallbladder, they cause no discomfort.

The pain usually occurs in the pit of the stomach or the upper right side of the abdomen and radiates to the upper right side of the back. It usually begins one to three hours after a meal and persists for several hours. It may be accompanied by nausea and vomiting.

What you can do

The greatest risk factors for gallbladder disease are eating a high-calorie, high-fat diet (which increases bile production), obesity and extreme dieting. Avoid fatty foods and overeating to help prevent a gallbladder attack.

see *Know What To Do*, p. 267

4

Kidney stones

A common disorder

Kidney stones are usually chronic, most often affecting adults between the ages of 30 and 40. They vary in size from microscopic to several centimeters in diameter. Most are made of calcium.

Note your symptoms

- Severe pain in the *flank* (the area between the last rib and the hip) and/or pubic region
- Nausea, vomiting (usually with severe pain) or abdominal bloating are common.
- Pain traveling along the urinary tract and into the genitalia, as the stone passes out of the body
- Chills, fever, frequent or difficult urination are less common.

What you can do

Kidney stones cannot be "cured" by self-care, but increasing fluids by three to five quarts per day and making some dietary modifications (ask your doctor for recommendations) reduce recurrences in many people. Carefully taking any prescription medication will also help (see *Using Medications*, p. 362).

Final notes

Most kidney stones will pass spontaneously, requiring only fluids and a pain reliever, with no further treatment. Medication may be prescribed to help dissolve existing stones and prevent new ones. For a small percentage of kidney stones, additional medical treatment may be required.

see *Know What To Do*, p. 267

know
WHAT TO DO

Abdominal pain
DO THESE APPLY:

- Chest, back or abdominal pain, especially if associated with shortness of breath, sweating or extreme paleness
- Jaundice, fever or persistent vomiting
- Abdominal pain and vomiting, especially if persistent, unusually forceful, or vomiting bright red blood or what looks like coffee grounds
- Unable to urinate and disabling pain

  see *Kidney Stones*, p. 266

- Abdominal pain is severe or is associated with chills, fever, rapid pulse, constipation, weakness or fatigue, or a sickly appearance
- Deep red (maroon), black or tar-like stools

YES

EMERGENCY ASSISTANCE

SEEK EMERGENCY CARE

NO

- Moderate to severe abdominal pain and you sustained a recent injury or blow to the abdomen
- Abdominal pain persists for more than 24 hours
- Fever, back pain, or you see bloody urine and/or symptoms are suggestive of kidney stones
- Symptoms are suggestive of appendicitis

YES

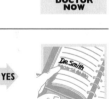

CALL DOCTOR NOW

NO

- Abdominal pain leads to a sustained loss of appetite or weight loss
- You have been diagnosed with gallstones and an "episode" persists for longer than three hours

YES

CALL DOCTOR

NO
---

see *What You Can Do, Appendicitis*

see *What You Can Do, Gallbladder Disease*

see *What You Can Do, Kidney Stones*

APPLY SELF-CARE

MUSCLES/BONES/JOINTS

Arthritis

Self-care helps manage symptoms

Arthritis means *joint inflammation* and refers to several diseases that
cause joint pain, swelling and stiffness. There are over 100 different types
of arthritis, but the majority of cases fall in one of the four listed on page
269. Most arthritic conditions cannot be cured, but their detrimental
effects can be limited with consistent self-care and medical support.

Prevention

While you can't prevent arthritis, it is possible to delay the onset and slow
the degenerative process.

- Avoid trauma, overuse and repetitive or jarring activities. Vary your
  exercise and activity schedule to allow changes in the pressure and
  stress on joints.

- Exercise regularly. Aerobic exercise increases blood flow to nourish
  joint tissues. Exercising with weights strengthens muscles that support
  and protect joints. Stretching and range-of-motion exercise helps
  maintain joint flexibility.

- Control your weight. Excess pounds place stress on weight-bearing
  joints such as knees.

What you can do

After arthritis has developed in a joint, self-care can help you maintain
joint function and decrease pain, swelling and inflammation.

- Take aspirin or ibuprofen to relieve pain and inflammation (follow
  directions and warnings on package). **NEVER give aspirin to
  children/teenagers. It can cause Reye's syndrome, a rare but often
  fatal condition.**

- Rest sore joints. If you must continue to put weight or stress on the
  joint, take breaks and rest.

- For inflamed, swollen joints, apply ice pack for 10 to 15 minutes every hour for two hours, then leave ice off for two hours. Repeat this cycle for 48 hours or until swelling is gone. For protection, place a washcloth between bare skin and ice. Do not use heat as long as there is swelling.

- If joint is not swollen, apply warm, moist heat for 20 to 30 minutes, three or four times a day. Follow heat with gentle full-range-of-motion exercises and gentle massage.

- When joint pain and inflammation subside, continue the prevention measures listed above.

- Become informed about your type of arthritis. Ask your doctor for self-care treatments specifically for you. Learn about resources in your community such as support groups, physical therapy, occupational therapy and stores that carry medical supplies.

MAJOR TYPES OF ARTHRITIS

Osteoarthritis	Rheumatoid Arthritis	Gout	Ankylosing Spondylitis
Cause			
Cartilage in joints wears out (degenerates)	Membrane lining of joint is inflamed, but cause still unclear	Build-up of uric acid crystals in joint fluid	Inflammation in spine, other joints; thought to be genetically linked
Symptoms			
Pain, stiffness, swelling in joints, especially fingers, may improve with rest; bony growth spurs can occur	Pain, stiffness, swelling in joints, with low-grade fever; doesn't subside with rest	Pain, stiffness, swelling, especially in big toe, ankle or knee	Pain, stiffness in back, neck and other torso joints such as hips
Commonly Affects			
Men and women, worsens with age	Middle-aged women most often	Men more often, aggravated by foods high in purines (such as organ meats) or alcoholic beverages	Men in their 30s, but stiff back can last a lifetime

For information about Lyme disease as a cause of arthritis, see *Tick Bites*, p. 158.

When to seek help

Although arthritis is a slowly progressive disease that can be managed well with self-care, there are three problems that require medical help quickly:

- Infection in a joint
- Broken bone near arthritic joint
- Nerve damage

Call your doctor if you have:

- Sudden swelling, heat or redness in joint(s)
- Joint pain that is severe or interfering with usual activities
- Joint pain that requires you to take aspirin, ibuprofen or any other pain reliever daily or frequently to ease the pain. **NEVER give aspirin to children/teenagers. It can cause Reye's syndrome, a rare but often fatal condition.**
- Pain upon motion of the joint, or limited movement
- Frequent joint pain and a history of ulcer or a bleeding disorder
- Joint symptoms and a rash or fever
- Inability to move or use joint
- Sudden pain in joint with numbness or tingling in limb below, back pain with numbness in legs, or loss of control in bowels or bladder
- Possible fracture (see *Broken Bones*, p. 75)
- Arthritis worsens or does not improve after six weeks of self-care (see *What You Can Do*, p. 268)

Neck pain

Many causes, slow to heal

Most neck pain is caused by straining the muscles or tendons in the neck and generally can be treated at home. But there are many reasons for neck pain. Neck pain caused by an accident or injury, such as whiplash from a car accident, can indicate a serious or even life-threatening injury to the spinal cord (see *Head/Spinal Injury*, p. 60). Chronic neck pain can be the indirect result of the aging process, resulting in degenerative disc disease.

Other frequent causes of neck pain are arthritis (see *Arthritis*, p. 268), meningitis or a pinched nerve.

MENINGITIS

Meningitis is an infectious disease that can be life-threatening. The classic symptoms are fever, headache and an extremely stiff neck — so stiff that you can't touch your chin to your chest. It can also cause intense muscle spasms in the neck (see *Know What To Do*, p. 273).

PINCHED NERVE

A pinched nerve can be caused by arthritis or a neck injury. The pain may extend down the arm or cause numbness or tingling in the arm or hand. **If you suspect a pinched nerve, call your doctor.**

What you can do

Environmental factors — your surroundings — can contribute to or cause neck pain. An uncomfortable mattress, a pillow that's too high, or an ill-fitting desk chair or work area all take their toll on the neck muscles.

If your neck hurts more in the morning:

- Try a firmer mattress on your bed, or use a bed board under your mattress to firm up a softer mattress.
- Use a pillow designed to protect your neck, or no pillow at all.
- Fold a bath towel lengthwise into a four-inch strip and wrap it around your neck. Secure with a safety pin while you sleep.

If your neck hurts more at night:

• Consider whether poor posture can be contributing to your pain. Walk, stand and sit with your ears, shoulders and hips in a straight line.

• Make any necessary adjustments to your office chair or work area.

• Keep elbows at a 90° angle for typing.

• Consider doing simple neck exercises every two hours, such as:

  - Sit or stand with an extremely erect posture to stretch the muscles in the back of your neck. Do it gently, repeating six times.

  - Squeeze your shoulder blades together gently six times.

  - Starting from an extremely erect posture, gently drop your head backward and repeat six times.

  - Gently drop your head backward, forward and side to side with gentle pressure from your hands, repeating six times.

If your neck hurts anytime:

• Aspirin or ibuprofen can help relieve pain and inflammation. **NEVER give aspirin to children/teenagers. It can cause Reye's syndrome, a rare but often fatal condition.**

• Apply ice pack for 10 to 15 minutes every hour for two hours, then leave ice off for two hours. Repeat this cycle for 48 hours or until swelling is gone. For protection, place a washcloth between bare skin and ice. Do not use heat as long as there is swelling.

• Heat from a heating pad (on the low setting) or shower may be helpful if muscle swelling is not a problem.

see *Headaches*, pp. 117 - 121, *Temporomandibular Joint Syndrome (TMJ)*, p. 207

Neck pain

DO THESE APPLY:

- **Neck pain associated with fever, headache and stiff neck**

  see *Meningitis*, p. 271

YES → **SEEK EMERGENCY CARE**

— **NO** —

- **Neck pain travels down one arm, or arm is numb and tingles**

YES → **CALL DOCTOR NOW**

— **NO** —

see *What You Can Do*

APPLY SELF-CARE

Back pain

Oh! My aching back!

Four out of five adults have back pain severe enough to interrupt their daily routine at least once in their life. A common and frustrating problem to treat, there is no quick, easy cure; recovery is slow; the pain often recurs; and prevention and treatment require life-long commitment.

Self-care is the major factor in preventing and treating back pain. Understanding the anatomy of the back and the most common injuries may help you decrease your risk of back pain and, if it occurs, quickly begin treatment.

Your backbone consists of 30 small, round, donut-shaped bones called *vertebrae*. Stacked up in an "S" arrangement (also see illustration on p. 276), the vertebrae form a protective tunnel for your *spinal cord*. The spaces between vertebrae are filled by *discs*, packets of tough cartilage with a jelly-like filling, that cushion and absorb impact. Your spinal cord, a bundle of major nerves, leaves your brain through the *vertebral tunnel* and sends branches around the discs out to the rest of your body. Large muscles and ligaments support the spine as it twists, bends, stretches, turns and maintains an upright posture.

CAUSES

There are many causes of back pain: muscles can be strained, torn or go into spasm; ligaments and tendons may be overstretched and sprained; discs become worn down, move out of alignment (*slipped disc*) or rupture (*herniated disc*); bones wear down or change, such as in arthritis or a fracture (see *Osteoporosis*, p. 319); and, occasionally, infection and tumors can be the sources of pain. In addition, back pain may not originate from the back itself but may be *referred pain* from problems in the prostate in men or reproductive organs in women, or from kidney infections or disorders in the stomach and intestines (see *Kidney Stones*, p. 266).

Pain from strains, sprains and minor disc damage is usually sudden, sharp and eases over two to three days with self-care. The sharp pain from a herniated disc or fractured vertebra usually lasts several weeks and

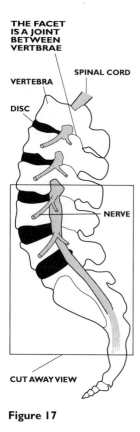

THE FACET IS A JOINT BETWEEN VERTBRAE

VERTEBRA

SPINAL CORD

DISC

NERVE

CUT AWAY VIEW

Figure 17

requires medical care. A steady ache is often a sign of disease, such as arthritis or referred pain.

Any back problem that causes swelling or a shifting in the alignment of the spine can put pressure on a nerve. Numbness, weakness or tingling are signs of nerve irritation. Nerves in the neck will produce symptoms in the arms and upper body, while spinal nerves in the middle and lower back affect the back, buttocks, legs and feet. Pressure on the *sciatic nerve* causes sharp, shooting pains down the back of the leg into the foot. Back pain can be constant or come only with movement.

Prevention

- Maintain good posture and keep the right amount of curve in your lower back:
    - Stand tall with your ear, shoulder, hip and ankle in a line. Do not lock your knees. Balance weight evenly on your feet.
    - Avoid wearing high heels.
    - Sit tall with your shoulders back and your lower back supported. Keep knees even with or higher than your hips. Avoid sitting in one position for longer than one hour.

- Use correct posture when lifting:
    - Bend your knees and lift with your leg muscles. Keep your back straight.
    - Never bend forward to lift. Keep the load close to your body.
    - Avoid turning or twisting while holding a heavy object.
    - Avoid lifting heavy loads above your waist.

- Sleep on a firm surface. Provide support for your lower back and under your knees if it feels more comfortable.

- Rise up from a prone position correctly. Rising is actually lifting your body's weight. Roll to your side and use your arms and legs to lift up.

- Maintain correct body weight. Obesity or a large abdomen can pull your lower back out of alignment.

- Exercise to maintain good muscle tone in your back and abdomen. Walking, swimming and biking are all good activities.

- Learn stress management (see *Stress*, p. 349) and muscle-relaxation techniques such as yoga.

4

What you can do

- Restrict activity. One or two days in bed may be needed in severe cases. Resume normal activity very slowly. Avoid any activity that puts stress on your back. Immediately stop any activity that causes or increases pain. Complete recovery may take up to six weeks.

- Apply ice or cold packs for 20 minutes every two hours for acute pain; decrease to 20 minutes twice daily once pain has lessened. For protection, place a washcloth between bare skin and ice.

- Once pain has lessened, take warm showers with water directed at the painful area.

- Take aspirin or ibuprofen to ease pain and inflammation (follow directions on the package). **NEVER give aspirin to children/teenagers. It can cause Reye's syndrome, a rare but often fatal condition.**

- Sleep on a firm surface. If possible, place a piece of plywood between the mattress and box springs.

- Support your back while sleeping. Place a pillow under your knees or lie on your side, knees bent and with a pillow between them.

- If back pain starts with no known cause, look for signs of a problem in another area of your body that may be causing referred pain.

- For minor muscle soreness in your back, apply heat for 20 to 30 minutes.

CALL CAREWISE FOR MORE INFORMATION

CareWise has excellent handouts related to first aid for back pain and progressive back exercises. A CareWise Nurse will be glad to send you information that meets your specific needs — just give us a call!

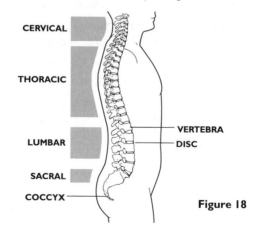

CERVICAL

THORACIC

LUMBAR

SACRAL

COCCYX

VERTEBRA

DISC

Figure 18

know WHAT TO DO

Back pain

DO THESE APPLY:

- **Sudden loss of bladder or bowel control**
- **Leg weakness or limited movement following a back injury**
- **Sudden tearing pain in upper back without muscle soreness**
- **Severe pain that goes down into the leg, groin or testes**

Keep still. Avoid movement. Slide firm support under total body if possible without moving.

YES →

EMERGENCY ASSISTANCE

SEEK EMERGENCY CARE

FIRST AID

APPLY EMERGENCY FIRST AID

— **NO** —

- **Severe pain in back and abdomen**
- **Burning or painful urination; brown, red or cloudy urine**
- **Recent abdominal surgery**
- **Taking medication to slow coagulation (blood clotting)**
- **Numbness or tingling in leg or foot**
- **Severe pain following a fall or accident**

YES →

CALL DOCTOR NOW

— **NO** —

- **Unexplained fever of 100.5° F, chills, nausea, vomiting or weight loss**
- **Chronic pain that does not improve after two weeks of self-care**

YES →

Dr. Smith

CALL DOCTOR

— **NO** —

see *What You Can Do*

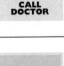

APPLY SELF-CARE

Shoulder/elbow/ wrist/arm pain

Self-care begins with prevention

Arm pain usually centers around the shoulder, elbow or wrist joints, more specifically around the soft tissues near the joints — such as muscles, ligaments, tendons and *bursae* (little fluid-filled sacs at the joints that help muscles slide over other muscles or bones).

BURSITIS

Through injury or overuse, the bursae can become inflamed and cause considerable pain. This is *bursitis,* which usually develops over several days (or less) from the time of injury or overuse.

Bursitis in the shoulder usually begins with a nagging ache that develops into more severe pain. Sometimes there is swelling at the tip of the shoulder.

Bursitis in the elbow may result in an egg-sized swelling at the end of the elbow.

Tennis elbow is a form of bursitis but is defined as any pain on the outside of the elbow and the upper forearm. It is sometimes the result of playing tennis but more often is caused by a repeated "twisting" motion of the forearm, wrist and hand.

For tennis players, using a two-handed backhand is one of the best ways of preventing this condition. In addition to avoiding the motion that started the painful problem, resting the arm is the best treatment.

ROTATOR CUFF TENDINITIS

This is an irritation of the tendons and muscles around the shoulder which tends to occur in baseball pitchers and those involved in racquet sports. Many times the pain is only felt when the arm is in certain positions. Swelling may be difficult to detect.

What you can do

If you experience bursitis or tendinitis in the arm, you may get relief from:

- Resting the part of the arm that hurts, and avoiding the motion or activity that causes the condition

- Putting ice or cold packs on the area. At the first sign of trouble, apply ice pack for 10 to 15 minutes every hour for two hours, then leave ice off for two hours. Repeat this cycle for 48 hours or until swelling is gone. For protection, place a washcloth between bare skin and ice. Do not use heat as long as there is swelling.

- Taking ibuprofen or aspirin. **NEVER give aspirin to children/ teenagers. It can cause Reye's syndrome, a rare but often fatal condition.**

- Maintaining strength and motion by gently moving the affected part through its full range of motion. The goal is not to let your arm get stiff.

CARPAL TUNNEL SYNDROME

Carpal tunnel syndrome results from compression of the *median nerve* (the major nerve) of the wrist. It is usually caused by continuous activities that involve repetitive use of the wrists and hands, such as using a computer keyboard or exposure to vibration (using a jackhammer, for example). The condition also can be the result of an injury to the wrist.

Hobbies that often cause symptoms include knitting, gardening, weight-lifting, painting and playing certain musical instruments. Medical conditions that result in swelling of the wrist — diabetes, certain thyroid conditions, pregnancy, arthritis and excessive use of alcohol — also may cause carpal tunnel syndrome.

Neglecting this condition can lead to permanent nerve damage and subsequent loss of hand function.

Note your symptoms

The pain associated with carpal tunnel syndrome is often described as burning, and can be accompanied by tingling, numbness or weakness of the hand, as well as shooting pain (particularly in the thumb and first two fingers). The pain is frequently worse at night and in the early morning. Unless an injury has occurred, the pain usually comes on gradually.

What you can do

If you suspect you have carpal tunnel syndrome, the first step is to identify the activity causing the symptoms.

If you discover that the cause is job-related:

- Try modifying your work or workspace. Adjust your desk, chair or keyboard height, or use a wrist rest.
- Avoid repetitive hand motions with your wrist bent.
- Take periodic breaks and stretch your hands and fingers.

For relief:

- Apply ice pack for 10 to 15 minutes every hour for two hours, then leave ice off for two hours. Repeat this cycle for 48 hours or until swelling is gone. For protection, place a washcloth between bare skin and ice. Do not use heat as long as there is swelling.
- Rest and elevate the hand and forearm above the level of the heart.
- Splint the wrist in a neutral position to immobilize it. The splint can be worn 24 hours a day if necessary, or only in bed.
- Hang arm over the bed if problem occurs while you sleep.
- Limit salt intake.
- Try using over-the-counter (OTC) anti-inflammatory medication, such as ibuprofen or aspirin. **NEVER give aspirin to children/ teenagers. It can cause Reye's syndrome, a rare but often fatal condition.**

Shoulder/elbow/wrist/arm pain

DO THESE APPLY:

• **Sudden arm pain accompanied by one or more of the following:**

- **Chest pain**
- **Shortness of breath**
- **Sweating**
- **Dizziness**
- **Restlessness**
- **Anxiety or panic**
- **Nausea or vomiting**

see *Chest Pain*, p. 218

• **Sudden arm pain in person with history of high blood pressure, coronary artery disease or heart attack**

YES

SEEK
EMERGENCY
CARE

NO

• **You experience signs of infection:**

- **Redness around the area or red streaks leading away**
- **Swelling**
- **Warmth or tenderness**
- **Pus**
- **Fever of 101° F or higher**
- **Tender or swollen lymph nodes**

YES

CALL
DOCTOR
NOW

NO

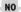
see next page

DO THESE APPLY:

see previous page

- **Numbness or tingling in fingers**
- **Suspect carpal tunnel syndrome and symptoms do not improve after one month of self-care**

YES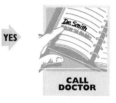

CALL DOCTOR

NO

see *What You Can Do, Bursitis* and *Rotator Cuff Tendinitis*, p. 279

see *What You Can Do, Carpal Tunnel Syndrome*, p. 280

APPLY SELF-CARE

Leg pain

A few possible causes

Most leg pain is caused by injury or straining the muscles and ligaments in the leg. Other conditions that cause leg pain are thrombophlebitis, intermittent claudication, shin splints and varicose veins.

THROMBOPHLEBITIS

Thrombophlebitis is inflammation and blood clots in the veins, which usually cause the leg to ache. This aching generally occurs after a period of inactivity, such as prolonged bed rest, taking a long plane ride or sitting through a long meeting. Sometimes a vein in the calf feels firm and tender, but not always. Swelling can also be difficult to detect.

The danger is a blood clot that can break off and go to the lungs. This is called a *pulmonary embolism* and is life-threatening.

If thrombophlebitis is suspected, call your doctor as soon as possible.

INTERMITTENT CLAUDICATION

When arteries in the legs narrow, the resulting pain is called *intermittent claudication.* The pain is "intermittent" because it's brought on by exercise and stops after a few minutes of rest.

When arteries narrow, blood cannot reach the muscles efficiently. During increased activity, such as walking, pain occurs. Older adults and heavy smokers are susceptible to this condition and are sometimes bothered even during such mild exercise as walking.

If you suspect intermittent claudication, consult your doctor.

VARICOSE VEINS

Varicose veins are a common and treatable condition in which bluish, swollen and twisted veins develop on the legs. They usually begin to appear on the back of the calves or on the insides of the legs when a person is between the ages of 20 and 40. They are almost always more unsightly than they are disabling. While they can't be cured, they can be treated.

Varicose veins are caused by long-term swelling of the leg veins near the skin's surface. This happens when leg muscles and the valves responsible for pumping blood back to the heart fail and allow blood to pool or collect in the veins. The veins then become distorted and swollen, particularly during prolonged standing. Feet and ankles may swell, and the calves and other affected areas may ache or feel heavy. These symptoms may worsen in women before or during menstruation.

In severe cases, the skin around the veins may itch and develop eczema (see *Eczema*, p. 130) or *ulcers* (open sores).

Varicose veins tend to run in families. They can be aggravated by prolonged standing or sitting, by being overweight and by numerous pregnancies.

What you can do

Varicose veins are common and usually mild enough for people to treat on their own. To lessen swelling and discomfort and prevent the condition from worsening:

- Walk regularly.

- Wear elastic support hose that reach all the way to the knee. Put them on after elevating legs for 10 to 15 minutes or as soon as you get out of bed in the morning.

- Wear shoes that support your feet well.

- Lose weight if you are overweight.

- Avoid standing or sitting for prolonged periods. If this can't be avoided, develop a habit of contracting and relaxing calf and leg muscles, knees and ankles several times a day.

- Avoid crossing your legs, wearing tight clothing or doing anything that inhibits the flow of blood from the legs to the heart.

- Never scratch an itchy varicose vein, since an ulcer can develop.

- If symptoms are bothersome, elevate legs above chest level twice a day or more for 30 minutes each time. Put pillows under your calves (not knees) so your ankles are higher than your heart.

See your doctor if, despite self-care measures, varicose veins develop ulcers, worsen or interfere with normal activities. Severe pain, tenderness and warmth in the area may indicate a blood clot. Call your doctor immediately and elevate the leg until it can be examined. If you suspect a blood clot, avoid massaging or rubbing the leg and avoid unnecessary walking.

SHIN SPLINTS

Shin splints is the general term used to describe leg pain on the front of the lower leg caused by overuse. It typically develops after a person who is sedentary overexerts, such as running three miles the first time out.

When the muscles and tendons that originate from the *tibia* (shin bone) become inflamed from repeated stress, pain results. Pain and tenderness are usually found on the front or the inside of the shin bone about halfway between the knee and ankle.

What you can do

- Rest your legs for at least one week after overexertion.
- Apply ice pack for 10 to 15 minutes every hour for two hours, then leave ice off for two hours. Repeat this cycle for 48 hours or until swelling is gone. For protection, place a washcloth between bare skin and ice. Do not use heat as long as there is swelling.
- Take aspirin or ibuprofen. **NEVER give aspirin to children/ teenagers. It can cause Reye's syndrome, a rare but often fatal condition.**
- When the pain is gone, do exercises to gently stretch the calf muscles.
- Wear high-quality athletic shoes, designed specifically for your sport of choice.
- Do not run for two to four weeks, then gradually increase speed and distance.

If symptoms persist, call your doctor.

Final notes

Severe, sharp pain one or two inches below the knee and tenderness in the shin bone are typical symptoms of a *stress fracture*. This tends to occur with an increase in athletic training where the legs are working overtime. Rest is the treatment for a stress fracture. Casts are not used. Complete healing takes four to six weeks. Call your doctor if you have severe leg pain.

see *Know What To Do*, p. 286

Leg pain

DO THESE APPLY:

- Deep pain or swelling in leg or calf

- Heat, redness or pain along vein

- Symptoms suggest blood clot: severe leg pain, tenderness, increased pain when walking, warmth, a feeling like a hardened cord in the affected area

  If blood clot is suspected, elevate leg and avoid unnecessary walking.

- Symptoms suddenly worsen

- Varicose vein bleeds when skin ulcer is bumped or scratched

YES

CALL DOCTOR NOW

— **NO** —

- Leg pain brought on by exercise; pain stops when exercise is completed

YES

CALL DOCTOR

— **NO** —

see *What You Can Do, Varicose Veins*, p. 284

see *What You Can Do, Shin Splints*, p. 285

APPLY SELF-CARE

Knee pain

Wobbly knees are more than nervousness

Knees are very delicate and vulnerable to injury. Ligaments and tendons that attach leg muscles and bones are easily sprained or torn when the knee is overextended, twisted or pushed from the side (see *Strains And Sprains,* p. 72). *Meniscus cartilage* (the crescent-shaped cartilage that is the shock absorber of the knee) can wear down, become too soft and tear from overuse or disease (see *Arthritis,* p. 268). The knee cap (*patella*) is a thin bone covering the front of the joint, and it can be broken or displaced.

Prevention

- Exercises that strengthen and stretch muscles and ligaments around the knee and upper leg are your best prevention. Walking, with warm-up and cool-down exercises, is one of the best choices (see *Staying Active,* p. 372).
- Avoid deep knee bends.
- Avoid running downhill rapidly or frequently.
- Do not wear shoes with cleats when playing contact sports.
- If you have arthritis, take your medicine — as directed.
- Wear stabilizing and supportive shoes. Avoid high heels.
- Avoid repeated, jarring motions on hard surfaces.
- Control your weight (see *Eating Right,* p. 373).

What you can do

- If knee pain occurs after an injury, rest and immobilize your knee. Start **RICE** treatment immediately (see *Strains And Sprains,* p. 72).
- Pay attention to the pain and avoid any activity that may cause or increase it.
- Use a cane to take weight off the sore knee.
- **DO NOT** put a pillow only under your knee at night; this may cause the joint to stiffen. Elevate the entire leg.
- If pain is caused by arthritis, see *Arthritis,* p. 268.

4

- Take aspirin or ibuprofen to ease pain and inflammation. **NEVER give aspirin to children/teenagers. It can cause Reye's syndrome, a rare but often fatal condition.**

know
WHAT
TO DO

Knee pain
DO THESE APPLY:

- **Severe pain following an injury**
- **Knee deformed or bent in an abnormal way**
- **Knee rigidly locked in one position**
- **Unable to bear any weight on knee**
- **Bone protruding or can be seen through the skin**

Immobilize knee. Elevate leg if possible. Apply sterile bandage if wound is open. Apply ice.

see *Broken Bones*, p. 75

YES ▶

SEEK
EMERGENCY
CARE

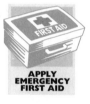

APPLY
EMERGENCY
FIRST AID

— NO —

- **Unstable, wobbly or very weak knee**
- **Popping sound, snapping or locking sensation during or after injury**
- **Pain in knee with swelling or pain in calf**
- **Knee is red, painful and feels hot when touched**
- **Knee pain with fever from no other apparent cause**
- **Severe knee pain even when not standing or putting weight on it**
- **Knee pain combined with another medical problem such as gout; or kidney, heart or liver disease**

YES ▶

CALL
DOCTOR
NOW

— NO —

see next page

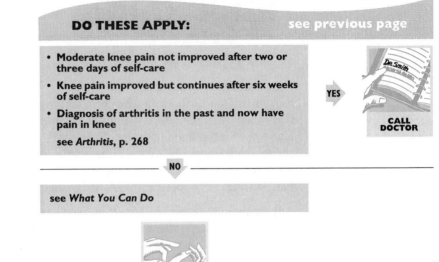

DO THESE APPLY: see previous page

- Moderate knee pain not improved after two or three days of self-care
- Knee pain improved but continues after six weeks of self-care
- Diagnosis of arthritis in the past and now have pain in knee

  see *Arthritis*, p. 268

YES

CALL DOCTOR

NO

see *What You Can Do*

APPLY SELF-CARE

Ankle pain

A very painful twist

Your ankle is a very complex, versatile joint. It is designed to keep your foot aimed in one direction while supporting the total weight of your body when you take a step. When it is not under pressure, the ankle allows the foot to flex and rotate. Problems develop when the ankle rotates while under pressure, such as twisting when you step; or the joint is injured by repeated high pressure, such as when you are running on hard surfaces or supporting excess body weight.

Ankle pain may be due to a sprain in one or more ligaments (see *Strains And Sprains,* p. 72), inflammation in a tendon (see *Achilles Tendinitis,* p. 296), a fracture in the ankle bone (see *Broken Bones,* p. 75), or damage to the sliding surfaces in the joint (see *Arthritis,* p. 268). Whatever the cause of your ankle pain, it is a message to relieve the pressure, rest the joint and provide support. Continuing to walk on a painful ankle without treatment may increase damage and delay recovery.

ANKLE SWELLING

There is frequently swelling with pain in an ankle injury due to damage to muscles and ligaments. Ankle swelling without pain or injury is often from the accumulation of fluid that has leaked out of the *circulatory* (blood and lymph) *system.* Fluid retention (*edema*) is caused by the build-up of excess pressure in the veins that forces the fluid out into the surrounding tissue.

Anything that interferes with the flow of blood from the legs back to the heart can result in ankle swelling. Some causes — including prolonged standing or sitting with pressure on the back of your legs, constrictive clothing such as garters or knee-high stockings, varicose veins (see *Varicose Veins,* p. 283), or a diet high in salt or sodium — can be helped with self-care. When ankle swelling is a sign of a more serious health problem — such as a blood clot (*thrombophlebitis,* see *Thrombophlebitis,* p. 283), heart failure, liver or kidney disease — treatment requires medical attention with individualized self-care.

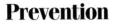

Prevention

- Wear shoes, clothing and sporting gear that fit well, have adequate support and are appropriate for each activity.

- Avoid shoes with cleats when playing contact sports.

- Wear stabilizing shoes. Avoid or limit wearing high heels.

- Avoid trauma, overuse or jarring activities such as running on hard surfaces.

- Exercise regularly. Always do warm-up (including range-of-motion) and cool-down exercises.

- Walk or do leg exercises a few minutes every hour when standing or sitting for long periods.

- Avoid wearing clothing that restricts blood flow. Wear support stockings.

- Control your weight and limit sodium in your diet if it seems to be a factor (see *Eating Right*, p. 373).

- Take all medications as directed. Check with your doctor before decreasing or stopping any prescription drugs (see *Using Medications*, p. 362).

What you can do

- If ankle pain follows an injury, start **RICE** immediately (see *Strains And Sprains*, p. 72).

- Avoid or limit exerting weight on ankle (use a cane or crutches if necessary). Listen to the pain. If it hurts, back off on activity.

- Support unstable or weak ankle with high-topped shoes or elastic wrap. Wrap ankle firmly, but not tightly, with elastic bandage. Start at the lower part of your foot, just above the toes, wrapping around the foot and then around the ankle in a figure-eight turn. Repeat figure-eight turns until the foot, ankle and lower leg (not the toes) are bandaged. Do not wrap too tightly or obstruct the blood flow. Loosen and rewrap periodically or if there is any tingling, numbness, change in color of toes or increased swelling.

- Do not wrap a child's foot; the risk of cutting off circulation is too high.

- Take aspirin or ibuprofen to ease pain and inflammation (follow instructions on the package). **NEVER give aspirin to children/ teenagers. It can cause Reye's syndrome, a rare but often fatal condition.**

- Elevate swollen ankles as often as possible with feet at least above hip level or preferably above heart level.

- When pain decreases, gently exercise ankle a few times a day:
  - Sit with leg hanging freely and gently; move foot up and down, in and out.
  - As ankle becomes stronger, support it with elastic wrap and walk on tiptoes, then on heels, to stretch and strengthen the joint.
  - Gradually increase the duration and frequency of exercise periods.

know
WHAT
TO DO

Ankle pain
DO THESE APPLY:

- **Bone protruding or can be seen through torn skin**
- **Ankle appears to be twisted, out of joint, or bent in an abnormal position**
- **Severe pain following a serious injury to ankle**

Immobilize ankle. Elevate leg if possible. Apply sterile bandage if wound is open. Apply ice. For protection, place a washcloth between bare skin and ice.

see *Broken Bones, p. 75*

YES ⟶

EMERGENCY ASSISTANCE
SEEK EMERGENCY CARE

FIRST AID
APPLY EMERGENCY FIRST AID

NO

- **Injury to ankle and severe pain even when not bearing weight**
- **Ankle unstable following injury with immediate pain and sound of snapping or sensation of tearing**
- **Ankle unable to bear weight for 24 hours or longer**
- **Swollen ankle with chronic kidney, heart or liver disease**
- **Ankle painful, red and warm to touch or fever of 101° F**

YES ⟶

CALL DOCTOR NOW

NO

see next page

DO THESE APPLY: see previous page

- Ankle pain and difficulty bearing weight for 72 hours or longer
- Ankle pain and swelling or discomfort in other joints

YES

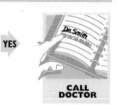

CALL DOCTOR

NO

see *What You Can Do*

APPLY SELF-CARE

Heel pain

Stress and trauma take their toll

Most heel pain is due to injury from repeated stress and trauma to the tissues that connect the bones of the feet and lower leg. These tissues bear your total body weight; are pulled in steps, twists and turns; are pounded in activities such as running and jogging; and often are stuffed into poorly fitting shoes with inadequate support. Is it any wonder that they sometimes hurt?

There are three primary causes of heel pain:

PLANTAR FASCIITIS

The *plantar fascia* is a tough band of tissue that stretches from your heel bone to the ball of your foot. It can become inflamed when it is over-stretched or torn by feet that flatten or roll inward with walking; feet with high arches; excessive running or sudden turning.

Shoes that fit improperly, offer inadequate support, or have soles that are too stiff or thin increase your risk of plantar fasciitis. This pain is usually felt in small spots just behind the ball of your foot, right in front of your heel or along either side of the sole. There may be some swelling in the painful areas. Repeated plantar fasciitis or extreme overstretching can lead to the development of calcified fascia splinters or *bone spurs* in the area.

BURSITIS

Bursae (*bursa* for one) are little fluid-filled sacs at the joints that help muscles slide over other muscles or bones. The *calcaneal bursae* surround the back and underside of the heel. Inflammation is most often due to pressure from shoes or landing hard on the heel. Pain and swelling are felt directly underneath or on the back of the heel.

ACHILLES TENDINITIS

The *Achilles tendon* is an elastic, fibrous band that attaches the muscles in the calf of your leg to your heel bone. Inflammation can be from shortening and lack of flexibility in the tendon, repeated hard contact or pounding of the foot, or unstable stepping or turning of the foot.

These factors often result from wearing shoes with high heels, inadequate support or shock absorption in the heel, insufficient warm-up and stretching prior to exercising, exercising on hard surfaces, and turning the foot as it strikes the ground. The pain of Achilles tendinitis can be sharp, a burning sensation, or a dull ache in the lower back of the leg and heel.

Prevention

- Wear shoes that fit properly and have adequate arch support; flexible, well-padded soles; and sufficient padding in the heel cup.
- Remember to stretch and warm up before exercising, including prolonged walking on hard surfaces (see *Staying Active*, p. 372).
- Ease pressure areas with moleskin patches.
- Wear footwear appropriate to the sport or exercise.
- Maintain normal weight.

What you can do

- Rest the area. Stop or decrease any activity that causes heel pain.
- Apply ice pack for 10 to 15 minutes every hour for two hours, then leave ice off for two hours. Repeat this cycle for 48 hours or until swelling is gone. For protection, place a washcloth between bare skin and ice. Do not use heat as long as there is swelling.
- Take aspirin or ibuprofen to ease pain and inflammation (follow directions on the package). **NEVER give aspirin to children/ teenagers. It can cause Reye's syndrome, a rare but often fatal condition.**
- Wear extra padding in shoes to protect and support tender area.
- Try slow, gentle stretching of the back of the leg for Achilles tendinitis; stop if pain starts or increases.

know
WHAT
TO DO

Heel pain

DO THESE APPLY:

- **Pain in back of leg or heel and unable to lift foot or walk**
- **Severe pain with redness and swelling**
- **Severe heel pain and fever with no apparent cause**

Apply ice pack. For protection, place a washcloth between bare skin and ice. Do not put weight on foot.

YES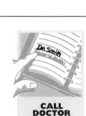

**CALL
DOCTOR
NOW**

NO

- **Pain is worsening or has not improved after four weeks of self-care**

YES

**CALL
DOCTOR**

NO

see *What You Can Do*

**APPLY
SELF-CARE**

Foot pain

When the shoe doesn't fit

Most foot pain is caused by shoes that do not fit well. Problems can be easily prevented and usually respond to self-care.

MORTON'S NEUROMA

Morton's neuroma is swelling in one of the nerves that supplies sensation to the front half of your foot and toes. These nerves run parallel along the five long bones in your foot and end in the toes. Tight-fitting shoes squeeze the bones together and pinch the nerve. This pressure causes swelling with intense pain in the ball of the foot and numbness between the toes.

PLANTAR WARTS

Warts are caused by a virus and usually appear on the surface of the skin. A *plantar wart* appears on the ball of the foot and grows inward so it feels like you are stepping on a pebble. This wart looks like an area of thick skin with small black dots scattered throughout and a center core beneath the surface. Unfortunately, they tend to recur (see *Warts*, p. 150; *Skin Symptoms*, p. 127).

CALLUSES

Calluses are hard, thickened layers of dead skin caused by friction. They often follow blisters and are a result of the skin thickening to protect an area against ongoing pressure. The ball of the foot is a very common site for calluses, especially if you wear high heels. Calluses can also occur on hands, fingers, toes or anywhere friction occurs.

Prevention

- Wear shoes that fit correctly. Avoid shoes that are too tight or loose, or that rub or slip.

- Wear high heels as little as possible. If unavoidable, alternate with pairs of shoes that have lower heels.

- Ease pressure areas with moleskin patches (available at drugstores).

- Limit your risk of contracting or spreading a foot virus by wearing slippers or bath shoes and avoiding going barefoot.

What you can do

- Take aspirin or ibuprofen to ease pain and inflammation (follow directions on the package). **NEVER give aspirin to children/ teenagers. It can cause Reye's syndrome, a rare but often fatal condition.**

- For calluses, soak your feet in warm water for 15 minutes, then rub the area with a pumice stone to remove thickened skin. Follow treatment by applying a moisturizing lotion. Repeat process daily until calluses disappear.

- Warts and calluses can be removed with an adhesive patch containing 40% salicylic acid, which is available at most drugstores. Put the patch on the affected area at night after soaking your foot. Remove it in the morning and rub off the whitened skin. Protect with a mole-skin patch.

know
WHAT TO DO

Foot pain
DO THESE APPLY:

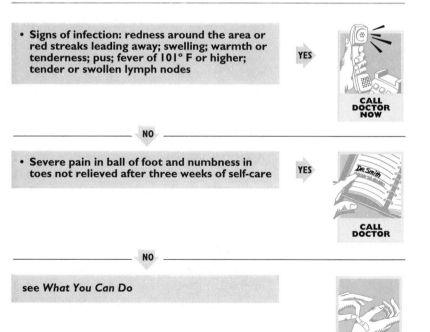

- **Signs of infection: redness around the area or red streaks leading away; swelling; warmth or tenderness; pus; fever of 101° F or higher; tender or swollen lymph nodes**

YES → CALL DOCTOR NOW

NO

- **Severe pain in ball of foot and numbness in toes not relieved after three weeks of self-care**

YES → CALL DOCTOR

NO

see *What You Can Do*

APPLY SELF-CARE

Toe pain

Small but mighty painful

Although toes are small, they contain many bones, ligaments, tendons and joints. In addition to being susceptible to all the diseases and injuries that occur in larger joints and bones, toes are often pinched, stubbed, and jammed, and have things dropped on them. What's more, they usually receive very little attention and care *until* they hurt.

BUNIONS

A *bunion* is swelling of the joint at the base of the big toe. The toe turns inward toward the other toes and may even overlap. This forces the joint outward, causing it to rub against shoes. Thick skin forms in the pressure area and, if the pressure is not relieved, a bony spur develops. The deformed joint often becomes inflamed and very painful.

CORNS

Corns are hard, thickened areas of skin caused by pressure from under the skin surface. The most common site for a corn is the top of toes where the tissue is squeezed between the bones in the toe and tight-fitting shoes. Corns are usually yellow with a clear core and may become soft, moist or red.

HAMMER TOES

A toe that bends up permanently at the middle joint is called a *hammer toe.* This condition is usually caused by wearing shoes that are too tight or narrow. The tendency to develop hammer toes is inherited.

INGROWN TOENAILS

When the edge of a toenail grows out into the soft flesh surrounding the nail bed, there is usually inflammation, swelling, pain and a high risk of infection. *Ingrown toenails* are caused by trimming the sides of the toenail too short, wearing shoes that are too tight, or injury to the toe or toenail.

Prevention

- Wear shoes that fit properly and have good arch support. Low-heeled shoes with a roomy toe box are best.
- If there is a high risk of trauma or injury to your toes, wear shoes with a reinforced toe box.
- Cut toenails *straight across.* Do not cut or file down on the sides.

What you can do

- Relieve pressure over painful area by wearing shoes that are roomy or open.
- Cushion area with moleskin or pads to ease friction.
- Take aspirin or ibuprofen to relieve pain and inflammation (follow directions and warnings on package). **NEVER give aspirin to children/teenagers. It can cause Reye's syndrome, a rare but often fatal condition.**
- For corns, soak your feet in warm water for 15 minutes, then rub the area with a pumice stone to remove thickened skin. Follow treatment by applying a moisturizing lotion. Repeat process daily until corn disappears.
- Corns may be removed with "corn plasters," an adhesive patch containing 40% salicylic acid, which is available at most drugstores. Put the patch on the area at night after soaking your foot. Remove it in the morning and rub off the whitened skin. Protect with a moleskin patch (available at drugstores).
- For ingrown toenail:
  - Soak foot in warm water for 10 to 15 minutes.
  - Wedge a small piece of cotton under the corner of the nail to train it to grow outward.
  - Repeat process daily until nail has grown out and can be trimmed straight across.

see *Know What To Do*, p. 302

4

Toe pain

DO THESE APPLY:

• **Signs of infection in ingrown toenail: redness around the area or red streaks leading away from toenail; swelling; warmth or tenderness; pus; fever of 101° F or higher; tender or swollen lymph nodes**

YES

CALL DOCTOR NOW

NO

• **Chronic illness such as diabetes or circulatory problems**

• **Sudden severe pain in big toe and no previous diagnosis of gout**

  see *Gout, Major Types Of Arthritis*, p. 269

• **Severe pain interferes with walking or daily activities**

• **Big toe begins to overlap second toe**

• **Symptoms worsen or do not respond after three weeks of self-care**

YES

CALL DOCTOR

NO

see *What You Can Do*

APPLY SELF-CARE

WOMEN'S HEALTH

Menstrual cycle

What's normal can vary

When a woman knows her own body, she knows what is "normal" for her. Women's menstrual cycles can vary from 21 to 40 days from the first day of one period to the first day of the next period. Bleeding typically lasts seven days or less.

Changes in bleeding may be normal, as with aging, or abnormal (see *Uterine Bleeding*, p. 309; *Painful Periods*, p. 311).

Painful intercourse

Several possible causes

Intercourse should be a pleasurable experience, not a painful one. Painful intercourse, or *dyspareunia*, for women can be caused by:

- Attempting intercourse without sufficient vaginal lubrication
- Vaginal or urinary tract infections
- Vaginal irritation due to an estrogen deficiency related to aging, breast-feeding or birth-control pills
- *Endometriosis*
- *Vaginismus*, an involuntary contraction of the vaginal muscles with intercourse
- Scarring from surgical procedures, such as *episiotomy* or *vaginal hysterectomy*

Pain in the vaginal canal usually indicates a vaginal problem. Pain that occurs when the penis is already in the vagina suggests a uterine, tubal or other pelvic problem.

What you can do

- When the problem is insufficient vaginal lubrication:
  - Since women tend to become fully aroused more slowly than men, try more foreplay before intercourse — leisurely, playful massaging and caressing of the entire body.
  - For additional lubrication, try saliva, or water-based gels such as K-Y Jelly, Lubifax, Surgilube.
  - Avoid lubricants that are not water-based when using latex condoms.
- If the cause is recent childbirth or vaginal surgery, nonintercourse lovemaking may be the answer until the vagina has completely healed.

Consult your health care provider if you suspect vaginal irritation or infection, urinary tract infection, endometriosis or vaginismus (see *Pelvic Inflammatory Disease*, p. 313; *Vaginitis*, p. 323; *Urinary Tract Infections*, p. 325; *Endometriosis*, p. 312; and *Menopause*, p. 318).

Pap smear

This can be a lifesaver

Examination of the female reproductive organs (a pelvic examination) gives your doctor essential information about your gynecological health. One of the most important elements of this exam is the Pap smear, which tests for the presence of cancer in the cervix and may identify endometrial or ovarian cancer.

A *speculum*, a plastic or metal duck-billed instrument, spreads the walls of the vagina so that a scraping of the cervix and a sample of vaginal secretions can be taken.

These cells are then sent to a laboratory where a trained technician studies them under a microscope and assigns them one of five classes:

Class I: No abnormal cells (negative Pap smear)
Class II: Atypical cells caused by inflammation, infection or
   benign growths
Class III: Abnormal or premalignant (precancerous) cells
Class IV: Severely altered cells (likely to be cancer)
Class V: Indication of cancerous cells

Pap smears detect about 90% of cervical cancers, making them reliable screening procedures. Since cervical cancers are slow-growing, there is an excellent chance regular Pap smears will detect the cancer before it spreads.

How frequently you should be examined should be determined by you and your doctor. Age, lifestyle and health history all play a role. A Pap smear is recommended every two to three years by the American Cancer Society after two consecutive normal screenings, until the age of 65. After the age of 65, the screening interval should be redetermined by you and your doctor.

A woman should have her first Pap smear by age 18, or at the onset of sexual activity (see *Screening Guidelines*, p. 378).

Breast lumps

Early detection may save your life

About 50% of all women will develop a breast lump before they reach menopause. The vast majority of these lumps are harmless. In fact, 80% of all lumps that are *biopsied* (tested) are *benign* (not cancerous). But some lumps are *malignant* (cancerous). With early detection, there may be more options for treatment and a better chance to catch any cancer that may spread to other parts of the body.

Men can develop breast cancer, but it's extremely rare.

Although some risk factors for breast cancer have been identified, 70% of all women who develop the disease have no known risk factors. Having one or more of the following risk factors *does not* mean that breast cancer is inevitable:

- Over 50 years old
- Having a mother or sister who has had breast cancer, especially if the cancer was in both breasts or developed at an early age
- Early menstruation and/or late menopause
- Having a first child after the age of 30, or having no children
- A previous diagnosis of breast cancer

Note your symptoms

A mass in the breast tissue may be hard or soft and can have a smooth or irregular contour. The size can range from microscopic to quite large. While some lumps are tender or painful, most are painless.

Some women have naturally lumpy breasts (called *benign fibrocystic breasts*). Fibrocystic breasts will feel lumpy and tender, and several lumps will be detected. The lumps usually increase in size just before menstruation and then disappear for a while when your period (*menses*) begins.

Fibroadenomas are another common type of breast lesion, characterized by a rubbery, firm, smooth mass. They are most often found in women under 30 and are almost always benign. Surgical removal of the lump cures the problem.

What you can do

THREE-PART SCREENING PROGRAM

Monthly breast self-examination: By taking a few minutes to check your own breasts each month, you will become familiar with how they normally feel and will be able to identify changes. If you still menstruate, the best time to examine yourself is two to three days after your menstrual period has ended. If you no longer menstruate, choose the same day each month to do the exam (the first day of the month, for example). Follow the six steps on page 308. Call your doctor if you discover any lumps, discharge from nipples or have any concerns.

Professional breast examination: Most major U.S. health groups now recommend that women age 40 and older see a doctor once a year for a professional breast exam.*

Regular mammography: A *mammogram* — an x-ray of the breast — is generally recommended every one or two years, beginning at age 50.*

*If your mother or sister has had breast cancer before menopause, beginning at age 35 have annual professional breast exams and mammograms every one to two years on your doctor's advice.

FIBROCYSTIC BREAST LUMPS

Fibrocystic breast lumps do not require treatment. Most associated pain or discomfort can be relieved by:

- Using mild analgesics such as aspirin, ibuprofen and acetaminophen (Tylenol). **NEVER give aspirin to children/teenagers. It can cause Reye's syndrome, a rare but often fatal condition.**

- Wearing a larger or more supportive bra during the premenstrual phase

- Eliminating caffeine

- Examining your breasts on a monthly basis. This is very important because the presence of cysts may make it more difficult to find a potentially dangerous lump. However, women who have benign breast lumps are not at a higher risk for breast cancer.

Final notes

Call your doctor as soon as possible if you think you have a breast lump, have unusual nipple discharge or have unusual pain or tenderness in your breast. The call could save your life.

Breast Self-Exam

Make these six steps a monthly habit

IN FRONT OF THE MIRROR

1. Stand up straight, arms at your sides and visually inspect your breasts. *Check for discharge from the nipples or puckering, dimpling or scaling of skin.*

2. Clasp your hands behind your head and press your hands forward. You will feel your chest muscles tighten. *Check for any change in the normal shape and contour of your breasts.*

3. Press your hands firmly on your hips and lean forward. At the same time, move your shoulders and elbows forward. *As in step 2, check for any change in shape or contour that seems different from the way your breasts normally look.*

IN THE SHOWER OR BATH

4. Raise one arm and with your opposite hand, press breast firmly with your fingers flat. Make small circles, moving from the outer edge toward the nipple each time until you have worked your way around the entire breast. *Check for any unusual lump or mass, especially between the breast and underarm, including the underarm.*

5. Gently squeeze the nipple. *Check for a discharge.* **If you have a discharge at any time, call your doctor.**

LYING DOWN

6. Repeat steps 4 and 5 lying on your back. Slip a pillow or folded towel under the shoulder of the raised arm. This flattens the breast and makes examination easier.

Repeat steps 4, 5 and 6 for the other breast.

For information from the National Cancer Institute call 1-800-4-CANCER.

Adapted from the National Institutes of Health

Figure 19

Figure 20

Uterine bleeding

Determining if it's a problem

BLEEDING BETWEEN PERIODS

Most women do not experience bleeding or "spotting" between monthly menstrual periods, but some do. Women who have an *intrauterine birth-control device* (IUD) inserted are especially likely to experience occasional spotting.

The key is how heavy the flow of blood is — and how often. If the bleeding is light and occasional, there is probably no cause for alarm. If the bleeding is heavy or has occurred three or more months in a row, the cause should be determined by a doctor. Bleeding between periods can be a sign of some serious conditions, such as *fibroids*, certain types of cancers or an abnormal pregnancy.

What you can do

If bleeding is light:

- Use pads or tampons.

- Avoid taking aspirin; it may prolong bleeding.

If bleeding is heavy:

- Contact your doctor.

MISSED/IRREGULAR PERIODS

Pregnancy is, of course, the number one reason for a woman who is not yet menopausal to miss a period. Home-pregnancy kits are fairly accurate as early as two weeks after a missed period, and a blood test can determine pregnancy 10 - 14 days after conception.

A positive test response is more likely to be accurate than a negative response. Unless you have another menstrual period, it's best not to believe the results of a negative test until it has been repeated.

Other causes of missed or irregular menstrual periods include:

- Stress: Emotional or physical stress can cause irregular periods.

- Obesity or strenuous dieting: Although these may seem like opposites, they have the same result when it comes to missed periods. If either is severe enough, periods may stop altogether.

- Strenuous exercise: Women athletes often have irregular periods caused by hormonal imbalances. There is concern now that this imbalance may also lead to a loss of calcium in the bones (see *Osteoporosis*, p. 319).

- Medications: Some medications may cause irregular periods.

- Menopause: If you are in your 40s or older, menopause could be the reason for missed periods. During this time, menstrual periods may be irregular before they stop altogether. Your doctor can determine if your symptoms are related to menopause (see *Menopause*, p. 318).

- Some diseases, such as *hyperthyroidism*, can cause missed periods, but these are relatively rare.

What you can do

Try to determine why you may be missing periods:

- If your period is more than two weeks late and you've been sexually active (even if you've been using a birth-control method), have a pregnancy test to determine whether or not you are pregnant.

- Lifestyle changes may be in order if you feel the cause is obesity, or strenuous dieting or exercising (see *Getting And Staying Healthy*, p. 372).

- Recognizing stress as a factor may help you focus on the cause of the stress rather than on the symptom (missed periods)(see *Stress*, p. 349).

- Keep a good diary with dates and details of your periods to report to your doctor.

see *Know What To Do*, p. 314

Painful periods

Some possible causes

MENSTRUAL CRAMPS

Menstrual cramps are medically known as *dysmenorrhea*, a Greek term meaning "difficult and painful menstruation." Medicine has finally caught up with what women have known all along — that menstrual cramps are physiological, not psychological and not just imagined.

Primary dysmenorrhea is common and caused by contractions of the uterus. Elevated levels of *prostaglandin*, a chemical produced primarily in the uterus, is thought to be responsible for menstrual cramps and other symptoms. These symptoms may include nausea and vomiting, fatigue, diarrhea, lower back pain, headaches and — in severe cases — fainting.

Secondary dysmenorrhea is the result of an underlying disorder such as endometriosis, pelvic inflammatory disease or fibroid tumors (see *Endometrosis*, p. 312; *Fibroid Tumors*, p. 313).

More than 50% of all women have at least mild menstrual cramps, and about 10% experience severe cramping that interferes with their daily activities.

Some degree of menstrual pain is considered normal, particularly in the first three days of the menstrual cycle.

Symptoms lessen for some women after childbirth or as they get older.

What you can do

For relief of menstrual cramps:

- Over-the-counter (OTC) nonsteroidal anti-inflammatory drugs (NSAIDs), such as ibuprofen and aspirin, inhibit the production of prostaglandins and may relieve discomfort and cramping. Acetaminophen (Tylenol) may help some women. You may need to try different drugs at different doses to find effective pain relief. NSAIDs and aspirin should not be used by anyone with a history of ulcers, gastrointestinal bleeding or any bleeding disorder without consulting a doctor (see *Home Pharmacy*, p. 364). **NEVER give aspirin to children/teenagers. It can cause Reye's syndrome, a rare but often fatal condition.**

- Exercise regularly.

- Eat a healthy diet. Avoiding salty foods for a few days before menstruation can help reduce premenstrual bloating.

- Avoid coffee and alcohol, but drink lots of fluids.

- Try applying heat — including heating pads on a low setting or hot water bottles — or take warm baths.

- Try switching to sanitary napkins. Tampons contribute to menstrual cramping in some women.

- Consider changing your contraceptive. Some women find that intrauterine devices (IUDs) make menstrual cramping worse. A barrier method or birth-control pills may work better for you. Oral contraceptives decrease production of prostaglandins and can minimize cramps (see *Birth Control*, p. 336).

ENDOMETRIOSIS

Endometriosis is a common condition that occurs when *endometrial tissue* (the lining of the uterus) grows outside the uterus, typically in the fallopian tubes, ovaries or pelvic cavity. This tissue responds to monthly hormonal changes just like the normal endometrial tissue inside the uterus, resulting in inflammation, bleeding and pain. No one knows for sure what causes this condition.

Diagnosis is difficult because the symptoms are not the same in all women. Typical symptoms include pelvic pain, menstrual cramps, irregular bleeding and infertility.

Women whose menstrual periods become more painful than previously, with the pain occurring just before and at the beginning of the menstrual flow, may have endometriosis. Abnormal uterine bleeding, especially heavy flows, rectal bleeding and pain during sexual intercourse are also common symptoms.

See your doctor if you suspect endometriosis. The objectives of any medical treatment are to control pain and to improve or protect fertility. For mild to moderate cases, the common treatment is hormonal therapy. For more severe cases, surgery may be required.

FIBROID TUMORS

Fibroid tumors — or fibroids — consist of bundles of smooth muscle and connective tissue that develop slowly within the wall of the uterus. These growths are almost always noncancerous and can vary from the size of a pea to that of a grapefruit (the size of the entire uterine cavity).

More than 75% of women with fibroids experience no symptoms. When symptoms do occur, they may include:

- Heavy, prolonged or painful menstrual periods
- Frequent urination or incontinence
- Abdominal pain or pressure in the lower back
- Constipation
- Pain during sexual intercourse

These tumors can remain unchanged for long periods of time and often stop growing without intervention. On the other hand, fibroids have the potential to develop into multiple, fast-growing tumors, and — in rare cases — can be malignant (cancerous).

If you have symptoms of fibroids, call your doctor. Treatment can range from birth-control pills (to help control vaginal bleeding) to surgery. Sometimes just the tumor itself can be surgically removed (*myomectomy*), but in some cases a *hysterectomy* (surgical removal of the uterus) may be required.

PELVIC INFLAMMATORY DISEASE (PID)

Pelvic inflammatory disease is a potentially serious infection of the reproductive organs that should not be ignored.

Pelvic pain with a heavy or foul-smelling vaginal discharge and/or a fever of 101° F or greater are symptoms of PID. PID can cause chronic pelvic pain and infertility.

If you have more than one sexual partner, you are at greater risk of contracting all sexually transmitted diseases. Some of these can progress to pelvic infection.

Pelvic pain that begins shortly before or during a menstrual period is probably menstrual cramps. If there is any doubt, see your doctor.

see *Know What To Do*, p. 314

Uterine bleeding/painful periods

DO THESE APPLY:

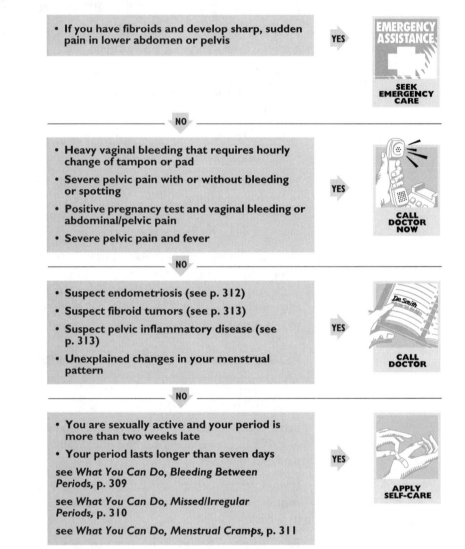

• If you have fibroids and develop sharp, sudden pain in lower abdomen or pelvis	**YES** → SEEK EMERGENCY CARE

NO

• Heavy vaginal bleeding that requires hourly change of tampon or pad • Severe pelvic pain with or without bleeding or spotting • Positive pregnancy test and vaginal bleeding or abdominal/pelvic pain • Severe pelvic pain and fever	**YES** → CALL DOCTOR NOW

NO

• Suspect endometriosis (see p. 312) • Suspect fibroid tumors (see p. 313) • Suspect pelvic inflammatory disease (see p. 313) • Unexplained changes in your menstrual pattern	**YES** → CALL DOCTOR

NO

• You are sexually active and your period is more than two weeks late • Your period lasts longer than seven days see *What You Can Do, Bleeding Between Periods,* p. 309 see *What You Can Do, Missed/Irregular Periods,* p. 310 see *What You Can Do, Menstrual Cramps,* p. 311	**YES** → APPLY SELF-CARE

Premenstrual syndrome (PMS)

A real and treatable condition

Premenstrual syndrome (PMS) is a medical condition involving both emotional and physical symptoms, which generally occurs seven to 10 days prior to menstruation. The precise cause of PMS is unknown, but it is thought to be caused by a change in hormone (*estrogen* and *progesterone*) levels.

It is estimated that at least 90% of menstruating women experience some form of PMS, but only about 10% have severe problems. Most women who suffer from PMS are between 30 and 45 years old.

Note your symptoms

Symptoms of PMS range from mild to almost disabling, and may vary in severity from month to month. They usually occur a week or so before menstrual bleeding begins, and end a few days after the period starts.

Symptoms may include headaches (including migraine), back and muscle pain, swollen or tender breasts, unusual food cravings, bloating, weight gain, diarrhea and/or constipation, extreme moodiness, depression, anger or irritability, anxiety and tension, insomnia and fatigue, lack of concentration or coordination, and diminished sex drive.

Asking yourself a few questions may help determine whether you are suffering from PMS:

- Do you have the same or similar symptoms every month?

- Do symptoms improve or disappear soon after menstrual bleeding begins?

- Do you have at least one symptom-free week each month? Answering no may indicate other problems such as endometriosis, vaginal or pelvic infection, or fibroids (see index, *Women's Health*).

What you can do

- Keep a diary for two or three months, recording the timing and severity of symptoms. This information will help your doctor make an accurate diagnosis and start an effective treatment program.

- Exercise regularly. Aerobic exercise — walking, riding a bike, swimming and climbing stairs — seems to work best to relieve symptoms.

- Adopt a diet that focuses on fresh fruits and vegetables, whole grains and a minimum of fats.

- Eat smaller meals every three or four hours.

- Limit salt (to reduce water retention).

- Limit sugar (to reduce blood sugar fluctuations).

- Avoid caffeine, alcohol and tobacco.

- Reduce stress in your life as much as possible (see *Stress*, p. 349).

- Try over-the-counter (OTC) medication (aspirin, acetaminophen or ibuprofen) to relieve discomfort. **NEVER give aspirin to children/ teenagers. It can cause Reye's syndrome, a rare but often fatal condition.**

- Talk about your problem with your family, friends or other PMS sufferers. Consider joining a PMS support group.

TREATMENT OPTIONS

Some women's symptoms are severe enough to require professional care. While no cure has been found for PMS, and doctors differ on its treatment, medications that may be prescribed to relieve symptoms include:

- *Diuretics* (medication known as water pills that increases fluid loss) to reduce water retention and bloating

- Antidepressant or antianxiety drugs to help ease emotional symptoms

- Progesterone — in the form of suppositories, injections or birth-control pills — to treat mood swings and other symptoms

Final notes

The best defense against PMS is to learn as much as you can about the condition and how it affects you, then begin experimenting with ways to manage and minimize the symptoms. Within a few months, chances are you'll notice that your symptoms have improved.

know
WHAT TO DO

PMS

DO THESE APPLY:

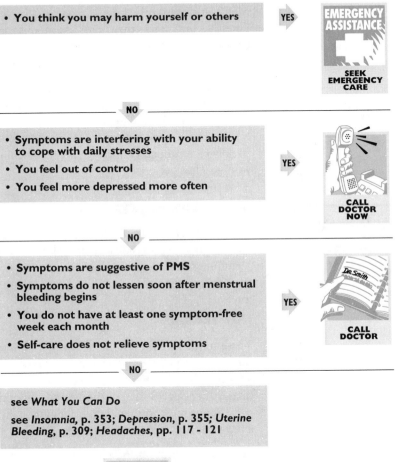

- **You think you may harm yourself or others** → YES → **EMERGENCY ASSISTANCE** / **SEEK EMERGENCY CARE**

NO

- **Symptoms are interfering with your ability to cope with daily stresses**
- **You feel out of control**
- **You feel more depressed more often**

→ YES → **CALL DOCTOR NOW**

NO

- **Symptoms are suggestive of PMS**
- **Symptoms do not lessen soon after menstrual bleeding begins**
- **You do not have at least one symptom-free week each month**
- **Self-care does not relieve symptoms**

→ YES → **CALL DOCTOR**

NO

see *What You Can Do*

see *Insomnia*, p. 353; *Depression*, p. 355; *Uterine Bleeding*, p. 309; *Headaches*, pp. 117 - 121

APPLY SELF-CARE

Menopause

The "change of life"

Menopause, also called the "change of life," is a natural event — not an illness — that marks the end of a woman's menstrual cycles and her ability to have children. It occurs for most women between the ages of 47 and 55, when production of the female hormone *estrogen* begins to decline.

Menopause can last a few months or several years, and it is considered complete when a woman has not menstruated for a full year. Menopause eliminates the need for any form of contraception, although doctors usually recommend continuing birth control until one year after a woman's last period.

What you can do

IRREGULAR PERIODS

Menstrual periods usually become lighter — but can become heavier — and irregular before they stop completely. Keep a written record, including dates, of your periods in case you need to discuss them with your doctor.

HOT FLASHES

These sudden feelings of intense heat, accompanied by sweating and flushing, normally last a few minutes. They are most common at night — although they can occur any time. Hormone imbalance caused by menopause can result in insomnia and subsequent fatigue (see *Insomnia*, p. 353). For most women, hot flashes gradually decrease over a period of a few years and eventually disappear.

To manage symptoms of hot flashes:

- Wear loose, lightweight clothing — preferably in layers — that can be easily removed.

- Drink plenty of fluids. Avoid caffeine and alcohol if they seem to bring on hot flashes.

- Exercise regularly to help stabilize your hormones and prevent insomnia.

VAGINAL DRYNESS

Estrogen helps stimulate the production of natural lubricants in the vagina, so the loss of estrogen can result in vaginal dryness — which can make intercourse painful and lead to *vaginitis* and an increased urge to urinate (see *Vaginitis*, p. 323).

Lubricants that provide relief for many women include water-based gels (K-Y Jelly, Lubifax, Surgilube). Do not use Vaseline or other petroleum-based products. In addition, many women find that regular sexual activity decreases problems with soreness during intercourse.

MOOD SWINGS

Hormonal and physical changes related to menopause may result in moodiness, depression, lethargy and nervousness. The best approach is to try to understand that this as a normal part of menopause and to be as accepting of yourself — and your moods — as possible.

OSTEOPOROSIS

The thinning of bones (*osteoporosis*) that is caused by reduced estrogen levels results in weakened bones that are easily broken. (This silent disease usually has no symptoms and goes undiagnosed until a bone suddenly breaks.) You are more likely to be a candidate for osteoporosis if you are Asian or white, have a slender body frame, are inactive and have a family history of the disease. Women who smoke or drink are also at greater risk.

To prevent or reduce the effects of osteoporosis*:

- Get plenty of aerobic, weight-bearing exercise — walking, aerobic dance, climbing stairs — to keep your bones strong. (While swimming is an excellent aerobic exercise, it is not particularly helpful in strengthening weight-bearing bones.)

- Make sure your diet includes sufficient calcium (1,200 to 1,500 mg per day) to help reduce bone loss. Low-fat dairy products or calcium supplements are good sources, along with vitamin D, to help your bones absorb calcium.

- Don't smoke cigarettes and keep alcohol consumption to a minimum.

*Women at greater risk, begin these measures *before* menopause.

Treatment option

HORMONE REPLACEMENT THERAPY (HRT)

This treatment option is currently the mainstay for treating symptoms of menopause. For some women, the use of HRT offers protection against osteoporosis and cardiovascular disease by reducing and even reversing bone loss, and improving cholesterol levels.

In 1975, a link between developing endometrial cancer and estrogen replacement was discovered. In order to reduce this risk and gain the positive effects of estrogen, the hormone is given in smaller doses along with progesterone.

HRT *may* be the answer if you are:

- Having difficulty with symptoms of menopause
- A prime candidate for osteoporosis
- At risk for heart disease

HRT *may not* be best for you if you:

- Have a personal or family (your mother or a sister) history of breast cancer
- Have had recent uterine or ovarian cancer
- Have an active blood-clotting disorder
- Are experiencing undiagnosed vaginal bleeding
- Suspect you are pregnant
- Have liver disease (such as hepatitis) or gallbladder disease

The decision about whether to use HRT is a very personal one. You will want to discuss the pros and cons thoroughly with your doctor and make the choice that best suits your body and your lifestyle.

Final notes

SURGICAL MENOPAUSE

Surgical menopause is caused by the removal of the uterus (*hysterectomy*) with ovaries (*oophorectomy*). In oophorectomy there is a dramatic fall in *estradiol* (estrogen) levels, often resulting in severe and abrupt symptoms. To help offset these symptoms, estrogen replacement therapy (ERT) is generally begun immediately after surgery.

Menopause

DO THESE APPLY:

You experience even minor vaginal bleeding and:

- **You haven't menstruated in more than a year and aren't taking hormone replacement therapy**

- **You are taking hormone replacement therapy and experience any unexplained vaginal bleeding**

- **Menopausal symptoms become intolerable or interfere with daily life**

- **You are avoiding social contacts or otherwise are unable to enjoy yourself**

YES → **CALL DOCTOR**

NO

see *What You Can Do*

see *Breast Lumps,* p. 306

see *Depression,* p. 355

APPLY SELF-CARE

Vaginal discharge

Has many possible causes

Healthy women produce small or moderate amounts of odorless, non-irritating vaginal discharge that may increase at certain times during their menstrual cycle. Abnormal discharge is very common and has many possible causes — some that require a doctor's care.

Symptoms	Possible Cause	Know What To Do
White, cheesy discharge; itching; burning with urination	Yeast infection (candida, monilia) or other forms of nonspecific vaginitis	Apply self-care if you have been diagnosed with a yeast infection before and think you have one now (see *What You Can Do, Vaginitis*, p. 324); if symptoms do not respond to self-care in three or four days, call doctor
Frothy discharge that is profuse and white, grayish-green or yellowish; vaginal burning and itching; may have urinary-related symptoms (see *Urinary Tract Infections*, p. 325)	Trichomonas, a form of vaginitis and urinary tract infection, is most often sexually transmitted; it can also be spread via damp towels, bathing suits and — theoretically — toilet seats	Call doctor now; if diagnosed with trichomonas, alert sex partner(s) and encourage them to see a doctor; abstain from all sexual intercourse until you no longer have symptoms (see *Urinary Tract Infections*, p. 325)
Murky white, gray or yellowish discharge; distinct "fishy" odor; itching	Bacterial vaginosis or nonspecific vaginitis	May go away on its own; apply self-care for vaginitis (see *What You Can Do, Vaginitis*, p. 324); call doctor if symptoms do not improve in three or four days
Vaginal discharge accompanied by severe lower abdominal pain, fever or recurrent or significant amounts of bloody discharge between periods	May indicate serious conditions ranging from gonorrhea to ectopic pregnancy	Call doctor now (see *Sexually Transmitted Diseases*, p. 339)

Symptoms	Possible Cause	Know What To Do
Discharge in young girl before puberty, or in postmenopausal woman who is not on hormone replacement therapy	May indicate other problems	Call doctor

VAGINITIS IS COMMON CAUSE

Abnormal vaginal discharge is the hallmark symptom of *vaginitis*, which can be the result of stress, antibiotics (that kill protective bacteria), use of birth-control pills, or excessive douching. It can also be transmitted through sexual intercourse. If you are pregnant or have diabetes, you are especially susceptible.

In addition to vaginal discharge, symptoms of vaginitis may include burning and itching, general pelvic discomfort, pain during intercourse, and painful or more frequent urination.

Prevention

- Wear cotton underpants that allow for air exchange in crotch and thighs. Avoid tight-fitting pants.
- Avoid douching and use of feminine deodorant sprays and other perfumed products.
- Wipe from front to back after using the toilet.
- Change tampons at least three times a day during your period. Alternate with pads and be sure to remove the last tampon when your period is over.
- Make sure to remove contraceptive devices after appropriate length of time.
- If you are prone to vaginitis, consume more acidophilus milk, buttermilk, cranberry juice and yogurt with live cultures to help the vagina maintain its natural chemical balance.

What you can do

Some types of vaginitis can be treated with self-care if 1) you have been diagnosed with a yeast infection in the past and you suspect one now; and/or 2) you have minimal symptoms and suspect a non-specific vaginitis.

- For a suspected yeast infection, try over-the-counter (OTC) antifungal creams such as Gyne-Lotrimin or Monistat. (If you have never seen a doctor for a vaginal infection, consult your doctor before using these products.)

- Avoid intercourse — along with douches, spermicides, tampons and contraceptive devices such as the sponge or diaphragm — while you have vaginitis to allow time for vaginal tissue to heal.

- Try not to scratch the area. Apply cold-water compresses or ice packs to reduce inflammation and soothe irritation. For protection, place a washcloth between bare skin and ice. Warm sitz baths (sitting in hip-high water) may also offer you some relief.

- Call your doctor if symptoms persist or worsen after three or four days of self-care, or if you are unsure what is causing your problem or what you should do.

Final notes

In most cases, symptoms of vaginitis disappear quickly with treatment. However, vaginitis does tend to recur, and some women simply seem to be more susceptible than others. Complications can be avoided by paying attention to abnormal vaginal discharge and sensations, and getting prompt treatment.

If you experience burning and pain with urination and feel like you need to urinate more than usual, see *Urinary Tract Infections,* p. 325.

Urinary problems

Don't ignore early signs

Burning or stinging pain with urination, frequent or urgent urination, or blood in the urine may all be signs of an infection in the lower urinary tract or inflammation around the *urethral* opening (the urethra is the tube that carries urine from the bladder and out of the body).

URINARY TRACT INFECTIONS (UTIs)

Urinary tract infections are also known as *UTIs, cystitis* and *bladder infections*. They are most common among women, but can also affect children, infants and men (see *Men's Health*, p. 330).

Symptoms may include a frequent and urgent need to urinate, pain or burning sensation during urination, cloudy or foul-smelling urine, pain or itching in the urethra, pressure in the lower abdomen, and lower back pain.

Between 80% and 90% of UTIs are caused by *E. coli* bacteria, which are generally found in the digestive system. Because the female anus and urethra are very close together, bacteria can find its way from the anus into the urethra and bladder. Any irritation to the genital area (such as sexual intercourse or wearing tight pants) can increase the likelihood of developing an infection.

What you can do

To prevent UTIs and minimize infection once you feel symptoms coming on:

- Drink plenty of fluids (eight or more glasses of water a day). Cranberry juice also may be helpful.

- Avoid alcohol, coffee, tea, carbonated beverages and spicy foods.

- Wear cotton underwear, cotton-lined pantyhose and loose clothing.

- Women and girls should always wipe from front to back after using the toilet (to reduce the spread of bacteria from the anus to the urethra).

- Avoid sexual intercourse when symptoms are present. Try to urinate before and after intercourse.

- Empty bladder frequently.

- Avoid bubble bath or bath oil, especially when symptoms are present.

- Avoid frequent douching and do not use vaginal deodorants or perfumed feminine hygiene products.

- If your doctor prescribes antibiotics, be sure to take the entire prescription as directed to help prevent a relapse or recurrence (see *Using Medications*, p. 362).

TRICHOMONAS

Trichomonas is a form of vaginitis that is usually sexually transmitted. Symptoms include painful or more-frequent-than-usual urination, and a large amount of vaginal discharge that is offensive in odor and white, grayish-green or yellowish in color. The *vulva* may itch and there may be a burning sensation in the vagina with spotting of blood. The pelvic area may feel uncomfortable and swollen, and sexual intercourse may be painful.

see *Vaginal Discharge*, p. 322; *Men's Health*, p. 331

know
WHAT
TO DO

Urinary problems

DO THESE APPLY:

- Adult diagnosed with a **UTI** has chills, fever, *flank* pain (the area between the last rib and the hip) or nausea/vomiting — especially if symptoms develop rapidly
- Pain in the small of the back, just above the waist (may indicate acute infection of the kidneys)
- A child under 2 years of age does not urinate in eight hours, only urinates small amounts, or has abdominal swelling; is vomiting, lethargic or feverish

see *What You Can Do*

YES ▶

CALL DOCTOR NOW

─────── **NO** ───────

- Symptoms of UTI or trichomonas
- Symptoms not relieved 48 hours after beginning antibiotics
- Visible blood in the urine without any other symptoms

see *What You Can Do*

YES ▶

CALL DOCTOR

─────── **NO** ───────

see *What You Can Do*

APPLY SELF-CARE

MEN'S HEALTH

Genital health

Examine the penis and testes monthly

Three minutes of your time each month can go a long way toward early detection of infections and cancers of the penis or testes. Early detection is the key to early treatment and cure. (Cancer of the testicle is one of the most easily treated cancers if caught right away.)

Washing the penis daily, particularly under the *foreskin* that covers the tip of an uncircumcised penis, can prevent bacterial infection and reduce the risk of developing penile cancer. It's an important routine to teach uncircumsized boys by the time they are 3 or 4 years old.

Once males are in their teens, they should also begin examining their penis and testes each month for any changes that could indicate infection or cancer.

What you can do

After a warm bath or shower:

- Stand with your right leg on the side of the tub or on the toilet seat.
- Gently roll the right testicle between the thumb and fingers of both hands. Check for:
  - Hard lumps or nodules
  - An enlargement or change in the consistency of the testicle
  - A pain or dull ache in the groin or lower abdomen
- Repeat this procedure on your left side.
- Feel the *epididymis,* the spongy tube on the top and the back side of the testicle. Pain could mean an infection.
- Examine the foreskin of the penis and the head of the penis for anything unusual, including sores, warts, redness or discharge.

WHEN TO CALL YOUR DOCTOR

Testicular cancer spreads quickly — within a few months — so it is important to see your doctor to rule it out as soon as possible after you find any testicular lumps or nodules.

Also discuss an enlarged testicle, groin pain or any penile discharge with your doctor.

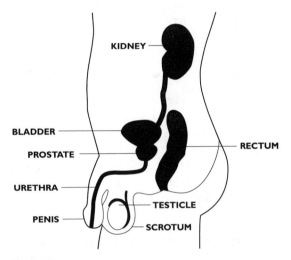

KIDNEY

BLADDER

PROSTATE

URETHRA

PENIS

RECTUM

TESTICLE

SCROTUM

Figure 21

Urinary problems

Detecting the cause

Problems with urination — difficulty getting urine started or completely stopped (dribbling), frequent or painful urination, decreased force of the urine stream, incomplete bladder emptying, blood in the urine — can have a variety of causes, ranging from a urinary tract infection to prostate cancer.

URINARY TRACT INFECTIONS (UTIs)

Urinary tract infections (also known as *UTIs*, *cystitis* and *bladder infections*) are most common among women (see *Women's Health, UTIs*, p. 325), but can also affect men, children and infants. In men, most UTIs are caused by obstructions or structural problems in the urinary tract. In men over 50 years old, the problem is often caused by an enlarged prostate gland that hinders the flow of urine out of the bladder and becomes the perfect breeding ground for bacteria.

Symptoms may include a frequent and urgent need to urinate, pain or burning sensation during urination, cloudy or foul-smelling urine, blood in urine, pain or itching in the *urethra* (the tube that carries urine from the bladder out through the penis), pressure in the lower abdomen, and lower back pain.

What you can do

- Drink plenty of fluids (up to several gallons in the first 24 hours after noticing symptoms). This can virtually wash the bacteria away. Water is good, and fruit juices that put more acid in the urine may provide additional relief (cranberry juice is best).

- Empty bladder frequently.

- If your doctor prescribes antibiotics, be sure to take the entire prescription as directed to help prevent a relapse or recurrence (see *Using Medications*, p. 362).

Trichomonas is most common in women but does occur in men. It is an infection caused by a single-celled microorganism called *trichomonas vaginalis.* The infection is most frequently spread through sexual intercourse.

Symptoms are uncommon in men but can include mild pain while urinating and discomfort in the urethra. In addition, there may be an unusual discharge from the penis.

Call your doctor now if you think you have trichomonas. If you are diagnosed with the infection, alert your sex partner(s) and encourage them to seek medical care (see *Vaginal Discharge,* p. 322).

PROSTATE PROBLEMS

The *prostate* (see Figure 21, p. 329), which produces some of the fluid in semen, is a donut-shaped gland that sits below the bladder and surrounds the *urethra,* the tube that carries urine from the bladder and out of the body. The three most common prostate problems are prostate infection (*prostatitis*), prostate enlargement (*benign prostatic hypertrophy*) and prostate cancer.

Prostate infection (*prostatitis)* is an infection of the prostate that may occur with a urinary tract infection as a result of bacteria traveling up the urethra. The prostate becomes swollen, constricting the urethra and causing urinary problems.

Symptoms include difficulty starting or stopping urination (dribbling), a strong and frequent urge to urinate while passing only small amounts of urine, pain or discomfort in the area behind the *scrotum* (the "sac" of skin that encloses the testes), low-back or abdominal pain, and pain and burning during urination or ejaculation. Fever and chills, a general ill feeling, and blood in the urine or pus-filled discharge are also possible.

The prostate can also become inflamed without bacterial infection (*prostate syndrome* or *prostatodynia*). The hallmark symptom is pain behind the scrotum or in the lower back. The condition is often related to stress or anxiety.

What you can do

Prostate infection requires a doctor's diagnosis and antibiotics, although self-care may be helpful as well; while prostatodynia may respond to self-care alone.

- Drink lots of fluids — both water and fruit juices.
- Avoid alcohol, caffeine, carbonated beverages and spicy foods.
- Ejaculate three or four times a week.
- Try warm baths or over-the-counter (OTC) pain relievers: aspirin, acetaminophen (Tylenol) or ibuprofen to soothe the pain. **NEVER give aspirin to children/teenagers. It can cause Reye's syndrome, a rare but often fatal condition.**
- Practice stress-management techniques (see *Stress*, p. 349).

Prostate enlargement (*benign prostatic hypertrophy* or *BPH*) is a noncancerous increase in the size of the prostate gland that appears to be part of the normal aging process; four out of five men between 50 and 60 years of age have this condition. It is not usually a serious problem, but it can become severe enough to compress the urethra and hinder the flow of urine as you urinate.

The hallmark symptom of BPH is *nocturia*, which is the need to get up at night to urinate. Other common symptoms include difficulty starting, stopping (dribbling) or maintaining the flow of urine; a decrease in the force or volume of the flow; or increased frequency of urination. Symptoms that develop as a result of the condition include increased fatigue, due to difficulty getting back to sleep at night because of nocturia; and mild dehydration (if fluid intake is decreased to avoid having to get up at night).

What you can do

- Avoid the use of caffeine, *diuretics* (medication known as water pills that increases fluid loss), alcohol and any over-the-counter (OTC) medications such as decongestants that have warnings related to causing urine retention.
- Take plenty of time to urinate. Sit on the toilet instead of standing.
- Do not limit fluid intake. Try to drink two quarts of water and other fluids throughout the day to help prevent urinary tract infections.
- Don't drink fluids after the evening meal. Empty your bladder before bedtime.

- If you have nocturia, leave a night light on and make sure the path to the bathroom is clear to decrease the risk of falls. You might prefer to keep a urinal at the bedside to avoid getting up at all — especially if you tend to feel dizzy or light-headed when you first get out of bed.

Prostate cancer grows slowly in many cases, remains within the prostate, and causes no health problems. In other cases, however, it can spread aggressively and become life-threatening (prostate cancer is the second leading cause of cancer death in men in the U.S.).

Symptoms include decreased strength of the urine stream, difficulty getting urine started or completely stopped, frequent and painful urination, hip or lower-back pain, and blood or pus in the urine.

What you can do

While prostate surgery is successful in many cases for localized prostate cancer, it can also result in impotence and urinary incontinence. As a result, men who are diagnosed with the disease may face a difficult dilemma: whether to undergo treatment and take the risk of side effects, or opt for "watchful waiting" and risk the possibility that the cancer will spread.

Watching and waiting — a process in which your doctor closely monitors your condition without treating it — may be appropriate if your tumor is small and appears to be growing slowly. (It is also common to do nothing in the way of follow-up for older men or for men who are in less than optimal health.)

If you and your doctor decide to watch and wait, you'll want to discuss how often you need to go in for checkups. Over time, if your doctor notices a steady increase in your prostate-specific antigen (PSA) level (a sign that the cancer could be spreading), it may be time to discuss a different treatment path.

Important questions to ask your doctor:

- What are my treatment options?
- What are the risks, benefits and possible side effects of each option?
- How will treatment affect my sex life?

- Will the treatment be painful, and if so, how will you treat the pain?
- Will I need to change my normal activities? If so, how and for how long?
- How often will I need to have checkups?

> If there is pain associated with urination or ejaculation and an unusual discharge from the penis, see *Sexually Transmitted Diseases*, p. 339.

know
WHAT TO DO

Urinary problems
DO THESE APPLY:

- **Inability to urinate at all**
- **Vomiting, back pain or severe chills (may indicate a kidney infection or kidney stones; see *Kidney Stones*, p. 266)**

YES → **CALL DOCTOR NOW**

—— NO ——

- **Symptoms of urinary tract infection or prostate problem**
- **Visible blood in the urine without any other symptoms**
- **Symptoms of UTI do not decrease after 48 hours of antibiotic treatment**

YES → **CALL DOCTOR**

—— NO ——

see *What You Can Do*
see *Painful Or Swollen Testicles Or Penis*, p. 335

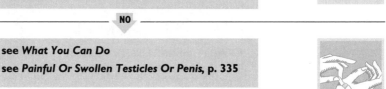

APPLY SELF-CARE

Painful or swollen testicles or penis

May require quick treatment

Pain, lumps, swelling or changes of any kind — even if they do not cause pain — in the testicles or penis may be a sign of a problem that needs prompt attention.

Possible causes include:

- Torsion — or twisting — of the testicle
- Internal damage to the testicle, due to an injury of some kind
- Infection of the lymph glands
- A recent case of mumps
- Accumulation of fluid
- A cyst or tumor

know
WHAT
TO DO

Painful or swollen testicles or penis
DO THESE APPLY:

- **Sudden, painful swelling of one or both testicles, without any injury to genital area, or pain accompanied by nausea and vomiting**
- **Sudden, painful swelling related to injury to genital area**

YES

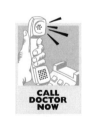

CALL DOCTOR NOW

— **NO** —

- **Swelling of one testicle**
- **Pain in testicles, swelling between ear and jaw, and fever (could be viral infection of glands)**
- **Painless swelling of the scrotum**
- **Unusual lumps or nodules**
- **Sense of heaviness in scrotum**
- **Pain or aching in groin or lower abdomen**

YES

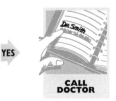

CALL DOCTOR

SEXUAL HEALTH

Birth control

Many options exist for family planning

Birth control is a personal decision to be made in the context of your own religious beliefs, health, lifestyle and financial issues. Today's options are varied — from age-old methods to forms that use the latest medical technology. All have benefits and risks that should be considered when making the birth-control decision that is right for you.

BIRTH-CONTROL METHODS

Method	Description	Effectiveness (success in preventing pregnancy after one year of correct use)	Risks	Comments
Tubal Ligation	Blocking of the woman's fallopian tubes so sperm cannot reach egg	99.5%	Generally not reversible; procedure causes minor discomfort	Surgical procedure performed by a surgeon; outpatient procedure; generally swift recovery
Vasectomy	Surgically cutting the tubes which carry sperm from testicles to penis	99.5%	Generally not reversible; procedure causes minor discomfort	Performed by a doctor; generally simpler and safer than tubal ligation; outpatient procedure
Contraceptive Injection (Depo-Provera)	Hormone injected into woman's arm or buttocks every three months which prevents release of eggs	99%	Irregular bleeding, weight gain, cramps; should not be used by women with certain medical conditions	Recent FDA approval; administered by doctor
Norplant	Hormone capsules inserted under skin of woman's arm which cause cervical mucus to thicken and block sperm from reaching egg	99%	Irregular bleeding, missed periods; should not be used by women with certain medical conditions	Surgically implanted by doctor; outpatient procedure

BIRTH-CONTROL METHODS

Method	Description	Effectiveness (success in preventing pregnancy after one year of correct use)	Risks	Comments
Birth-Control Pills	Pills taken orally by woman to prevent the release of eggs from the ovaries; contain hormones such as synthetic estrogen and progesterone	97%	Low potential risk for blood clots, high blood pressure, stroke, heart attack; do not provide protection against HIV (AIDS virus)	Must be prescribed by doctor; used by more than 200 million women worldwide; effectiveness linked to conscientious use
IUD (Intrauterine Device)	A copper wire device inserted in uterus; unit may secrete hormones; appears to prevent fertilized egg from implanting in uterus by causing inflammation of uterine lining	95% to 98%	May cause strong cramps, abnormal bleeding; can be linked to PID (pelvic inflammatory disease), which can scar the fallopian tubes and result in infertility; no protection against sexually transmitted diseases	Should be used under doctor's supervision; can pose risk if pregnancy occurs
Condom for Men	A thin, glove-like sheath which covers the penis to prevent sperm from entering woman's reproductive system; latex is recommended	88% to 97%	No side effects; greatest risk is incorrect or inconsistent usage; may cause irritation	Available without prescription; low cost; also reduces spread of HIV and sexually transmitted diseases
Diaphragm	Dome-shaped rubber cup that fits over woman's cervix to block sperm from entering uterus; must be inserted before intercourse	82% to 94%	Usually none; prolonged wearing for more than six to eight hours can lead to infection or possibly toxic shock syndrome, a sometimes fatal condition	Prescribed and fitted by doctor; should remain in place six hours after intercourse; can protect against some sexually transmitted diseases; best if used with spermicide
Cervical Cap	Similar to diaphragm: small rubber cup which fits over cervix to block sperm from entering uterus; must be inserted before intercourse	82% to 94%	Prolonged wearing can lead to toxic shock syndrome, a sometimes fatal condition	Prescribed and fitted by doctor; not as widely available as diaphragm

4

BIRTH-CONTROL METHODS

Method	Description	Effectiveness (success in preventing pregnancy after one year of correct use)	Risks	Comments
Periodic Abstinence	Abstaining from intercourse during ovulation, a woman's most fertile period, usually 14 days before the onset of menstrual flow	80%	No side effects	Dependent on ability to accurately chart fertile periods; not a foolproof method
Spermicides	Foams, creams or suppositories inserted in woman's vagina to destroy sperm before they can enter uterus and fertilize egg	Varies widely from 60% to 98%	Usually no side effects; can cause skin irritation; greatest risk is irregular usage	Available without prescription; low cost; more effective if used with diaphragm or condom
Withdrawal	Withdrawing penis from vagina before ejaculation of sperm	Very low	No side effects	Unreliable; small amounts of sperm-laden semen can leak out before ejaculation
Condom for Women	Sheath which lines woman's vagina to block sperm from reaching egg	Not known; likely to be similar to male condom	No known health risks; greatest risk is from incorrect or inconsistent usage	Recently approved by FDA; still little information available; most effective if used with spermicide; reduces spread of sexually transmitted diseases

Sexually transmitted diseases (STDs)

Safe sex is key to prevention

Most sexually transmitted diseases (STDs) can be prevented by following basic safe-sex measures (see *Safe Sex*, p. 347). AIDS poses special risks, including transmission by needles and from mother to fetus (see *HIV*, p. 344). Although genital herpes is an incurable STD, it can be managed with self-care and medical treatment (see *Genital Herpes*, p. 341). **Always consult your doctor for diagnosis and treatment.**

SEXUALLY TRANSMITTED DISEASES

Disease	Cause	Signs	Diagnosis	Final Notes
Chlamydia	Bacteria	General pelvic pain; frequent burning urination; discomfort during sexual intercourse; vaginal discharge	Pelvic exam and/or test or culture from the cervix, examination of tissue or biopsy	Treated with antibiotics; if untreated chlamydia can cause pelvic inflammatory disease (PID), infertility in women and complications in pregnancy
Genital Warts (HPV)	Virus	Small, fleshy growths in genital, anal or mouth areas; singular or in clusters	Physical exam	Cryotherapy, topical medications, surgical removal; genital warts often reappear after treatment

SEXUALLY TRANSMITTED DISEASES

Disease	Cause	Signs	Diagnosis	Final Notes
Gonorrhea	Bacteria	Men: mucous and pus-filled discharge from penis; slow, painful or difficult urination; Women: mucous and pus-filled vaginal discharge; vaginal itching; painful or burning urination	Physical exam and lab tests of vaginal culture	Untreated gonorrhea can lead to PID or cause arthritis, infertility and other serious problems
Syphilis	Bacteria	Painless sore on genitals, anus or in mouth two to four weeks after infection, hardening into a painless ulcer then disappearing; swollen lymph nodes, fever, and/or rashes four to six weeks after infection	Blood test, examination of fluid from sores	Untreated syphilis can lead to blindness, brain damage and heart disease

Prevention

You can prevent STDs by practicing safe sex:

· Always use a latex condom

· Limit the number of sex partners

· Have partners tested for STDs

· Avoid sex with infected individuals

see *Safe Sex*, p. 347

Genital herpes

It's with you for life

Herpes viruses can cause conditions such as chicken pox and *mononucleosis*. Herpes simplex virus type 1 typically causes fever blisters/cold sores on the lips and mouth. Herpes simplex virus type 2 causes genital herpes, which infects the genital and *anorectal* (anus and/or rectum) areas.

However, herpes simplex virus type 1 *can* infect the genital area, usually through oral sex, and herpes simplex type 2 can infect the lips or mouth. Once either virus enters the body, you can never be completely free of it (to avoid genital herpes, always practice safe sex; see *Safe Sex*, p. 347). But you can help limit the spread of infection and reduce the discomfort of an outbreak.

During the first outbreak of genital herpes, blisters turn into well-defined ulcers or sores, form crusts and heal in one to three weeks. After the first outbreak, many people experience periodic but milder attacks as smaller clusters of blisters appear and last up to 10 days.

What you can do

Although there is no cure for genital herpes, these measures can help relieve your discomfort:

- Five- to 10-minute sitz baths (soaking in hip-high, warm water) may be soothing and help promote healing.

- Apply cool compresses soaked in Burrow's solution, or gently dab herpes sores in the genital or rectal area with pads soaked in witch hazel.

- Use a hair dryer set on low to help dry up blisters.

- Try to reduce stress and anxiety (see *Stress*, p. 349). This can help prevent outbreaks.

  (Call CareWise if you'd like a brochure on stress-management techniques.)

- Nonprescription pain relievers (aspirin, acetaminophen or ibuprofen) usually help. **NEVER give aspirin to children/teenagers. It can cause Reye's syndrome, a rare but often fatal condition.**

- Wash hands frequently to prevent spreading the disease.

ALERTING YOUR SEX PARTNER(S)

You will have to tell your sex partner(s) that they have been exposed to the virus so they can be evaluated by a doctor, treated if necessary, and advised to continue checking themselves for herpes outbreaks. If you are hesitant to talk to your sex partner(s), ask your doctor for advice.

Final notes

Most people with genital herpes experience itching, tingling or burning in the affected area a day or two before blisters appear. Acyclovir is the drug most often prescribed for first-time outbreaks. Daily treatment does not eliminate the risk of transmitting the virus. Until all sores have healed, the herpes virus is highly contagious.

Avoid sex until all the sores have healed. Because the virus can be spread even when there are no apparent sores, always use a latex condom for your partner's safety. Even though infection can still occur if condoms are used, some protection is better than none. Genital sores from any cause increase the risk of HIV or AIDS. Always practice safe sex.

see *Safe Sex*, p. 347

know
WHAT TO DO

Genital herpes
DO THESE APPLY:

- **Signs of infection:**
  - **Redness around the area or red streaks leading away**
  - **Swelling**
  - **Warmth or tenderness**
  - **Pus**
  - **Fever of 101° F or higher**
  - **Tender or swollen lymph nodes**

YES ▶ **CALL DOCTOR NOW**

--- NO ---

- **Genital blisters for the first time; mild flu-like symptoms with fever, malaise, loss of appetite and swelling of lymph nodes (early medical treatment may greatly reduce symptoms)**
- **Small blisters develop within 24 to 48 hours on body where there was sexual contact**
- **Recurrent symptoms are severe or frequent or last more than two weeks**
- **You're pregnant and have, or have had, genital herpes**

YES ▶ **CALL DOCTOR**

--- NO ---

Avoid sexual contact during an outbreak and the period right before an outbreak.

see *What You Can Do*

see *Safe Sex*, p. 347

APPLY SELF-CARE

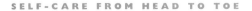

4

Human immunodeficiency virus (HIV)

It causes AIDS

The human immunodeficiency virus (HIV) causes acquired immunodeficiency syndrome (AIDS). If you test positive for HIV, you carry the virus and can infect others but may not have symptoms of the illness for some time. For adults, the average period from infection with the virus to development of AIDS is 10 years. After AIDS develops, death usually occurs within two or three years.

Some 1 to 1.5 million Americans and 5 to 10 million people worldwide are HIV-positive. For about a decade after it was recognized in the United States, AIDS primarily infected homosexual and bisexual men. Currently, however, the biggest increase in AIDS is among heterosexuals through intercourse. More women than men are becoming infected this way.

Note your symptoms

Some people experience symptoms of an acute viral infection within a few months after exposure. The symptoms typically last one to two weeks and resemble *infectious mononucleosis*: swollen glands, sore throat, fever, malaise, skin rash (see *Mononucleosis*, p. 174; *Swollen Glands*, p. 180). Years may pass before early symptoms of AIDS appear, including:

- Prolonged, unexplained fatigue
- Fever lasting more than 10 days
- Night sweats
- Swollen glands or rapid weight loss
- Persistent diarrhea, colds, unexplained dry cough or sore throat
- Easy bruising or unexplained bleeding

TRANSMISSION

HIV is spread by unprotected sexual intercourse, sharing needles or syringes with someone who has HIV, receiving contaminated blood or blood products, from mother to fetus during pregnancy, and from mother to infant through breast-feeding.

Prevention

You can prevent infection with HIV by eliminating risky behaviors:

- Limit your sex partners or abstain completely.

- Avoid unprotected sexual intercourse (oral, vaginal, anal). Always use latex condoms unless you are in a monogamous relationship and you and your partner have tested negative for HIV for six months or longer.

- Don't use intravenous (IV) drugs, or share needles or syringes.

see *Safe Sex,* p. 347

NOTE: HIV does not appear to be transmitted through saliva, tears, sweat or feces. Nor can it be transmitted through mosquito bites, donating blood or contact with inanimate objects such as toilet seats. An infected person who is coughing, talking or eating poses no risk of spreading HIV to others.

TESTING FOR HIV

- Do you suspect you have been exposed to HIV? If so, get tested immediately and repeat the test in six months. Continue testing every three to six months for as long as your high-risk behavior continues.

- Is your HIV test positive but you have no symptoms of AIDS? Schedule follow-up visits and tests with your doctor.

- Cooperate with your doctor and public health officials in identifying your sex partner(s) so they may be alerted to the possibility of exposure to HIV.

What you can do

There is no vaccine for HIV infection and no drug that is effective against the virus. Your best strategy for dealing with HIV is to prevent exposure by abstaining or practicing safe sex.

Final notes

Drugs that hold promise in slowing the development of AIDS complications include AZT (azidothymidine), ddI (dideoxyinosine) and ddC (dideoxycytidine). None of these are cures and all have major side effects. People who test positive for HIV often experience depression and job-security issues, as well as major social and financial challenges. For more information on counseling resources, contact the Centers for Disease Control AIDS hotline, 1-800-342-2437. **Always consult your doctor for diagnosis and treatment.**

For more information about Sexually Transmitted Diseases, see p. 339

Safe sex

The only defense against AIDS

Prevention is the *only* defense against AIDS and the *best* defense against other sexually transmitted diseases (STDs). There is no vaccine for HIV (the virus that causes AIDS). It's what you do — not who you are — that puts you at risk. Anyone can get AIDS.

What you can do

PREVENTION

- Eliminate your risk entirely by not having sex with anyone (abstinence) or by having sex only with a non-infected partner who has sex only with you (mutual monogamy).

- Unless you are in a monogamous relationship and you and your partner have tested negative for HIV for six months or longer (or have been in a mutually monogomous relationship since the late 70s):
  - Use a latex condom each time you have sex.
  - Avoid unprotected vaginal, oral and anal sex.

- Don't use "natural" skin condoms. Only latex condoms protect against HIV/STDs. In addition:
  - Always check the condom for tears.
  - Cover the erect penis with the condom before any sexual contact.
  - Keep the condom snugly in place until sexual contact is over.

- If needed, use a water-based lubricant, such as K-Y Jelly during intercourse. Avoid petroleum-based products, which can weaken the latex barrier.

- Get to know your sexual partner(s) before you have sexual relations, and limit the number of partners you have.

- Behaviors that are considered to put you at high risk for contracting HIV include having sex with:
  - Intravenous (IV) drug users, or anyone who has had sex with an IV drug user
  - Someone who has or has had numerous sexual partners

- Someone who has or has had an STD such as genital herpes, syphilis, gonorrhea or any open genital or oral sore

- Someone who has received a blood transfusion or blood products between 1978 - 85 and has not been tested for HIV

- Male or female prostitutes

- Homosexual or bisexual men

- Individuals with questionable HIV status

Final notes

Although sexual intercourse is the primary means of infection with HIV, it is not the only one. Infants can be born with the virus if their mother is infected, and HIV can be passed to children through breast milk from infected mothers. **Always consult your doctor for diagnosis and treatment.**

see *Sexually Transmitted Diseases*, p. 339

MENTAL HEALTH

Stress

Necessary — in moderation

Anyone who has been late for an important appointment or struggled with the family finances knows that stress is a normal and even useful reaction.

In stressful situations or emergencies, our bodies automatically increase production of certain hormones. This results in a rise in heart rate and blood pressure, a tensing of muscles to prepare the body for action, an increase in perspiration to cool the body, faster respiration to raise the oxygen supply, and a dilation of the pupils to improve vision. These responses, known as "fight or flight," were once vital to the survival of the human race.

Today, we're rarely in life-or-death situations, but our bodies still react to stress in the same old ways. This is particularly clear during times of major life changes such as divorce, death, illness, moving or changing jobs.

Note your symptoms

Stress in itself is neither good nor bad, but how we react to stress can have a huge impact on our well-being. *Anxiety* is one way to react to stress. Symptoms of anxiety include insomnia, inability to concentrate, tension headaches and upset stomach. Stress also can cause *depression* that might show itself as reclusiveness, irritability or pessimism.

Grief is a response to the loss of a loved one, job or something else dear to us.

In extreme cases of stress, such as war or natural disaster, *posttraumatic stress disorder (PTSD)* can develop. It's characterized by the persistent "re-experiencing" of the stressful event with flashbacks and sometimes hallucinations. Other symptoms include avoiding thoughts and feelings about the event, emotional withdrawal, insomnia, irritability and an exaggerated startle response.

What you can do

The physical symptoms of stress can be alleviated after you recognize the sources of stress. For example, if job anxiety is continually causing an upset stomach, you won't solve the problem simply by treating the stomach pain. The key is to find ways to minimize or manage reactions to stress.

LOOK FOR CREATIVE SOLUTIONS

- Would joining a carpool help reduce stress related to commuting?
- Would hiring a babysitter for a few hours a day help?
- Can home chores be rearranged or taken over by others?

CONSIDER OTHER STRESS-MANAGEMENT TOOLS

- Exercise regularly.
- Pursue hobbies.
- Talk things over with a friend.
- Cry if that helps you feel better.
- Try yoga, meditation or other muscle-relaxation techniques.

TRY TO KEEP THINGS IN PERSPECTIVE

- Let go of things that are beyond your control.
- Imagine the worst that could happen in any given situation, the likelihood that it will occur, and how you would handle it if it did.
- Consider whether you will even remember this event in a few years.

During extremely stressful situations, such as the death of a family member, taking time to experience your feelings of sadness and loss is an important step toward emotional healing.

Final notes

If you feel you can't cope with a problem, talk to a counselor, psychiatrist, clergyperson or CareWise Nurse. These steps might be particularly helpful if you can't identify the cause of stress but are having troublesome symptoms.

Seek immediate emergency care if you are thinking about suicide or doing physical harm to others. Call your doctor if you are turning to alcohol or drugs to relieve stress.

HYPERVENTILATION SYNDROME

Hyperventilation is when you breathe too fast. The result is that too much oxygen is taken into your system, and the carbon dioxide level in your blood is lowered. *Hyperventilation syndrome* is when this happens as a result of anxiety.

Hyperventilation causes you to feel out of breath and can bring on dizziness or numbness and tingling of the hands, feet and mouth. In severe cases, there can be chest pain, spasms of the heart muscles or even unconsciousness.

Most common in young adults, hyperventilation syndrome usually is found in anxious or nervous people who develop concerns about their ability to breathe.

Hyperventilation can also be a reaction to severe pain. The cause needs to be determined to eliminate the symptoms.

What you can do

If you know someone has a history of hyperventilating, offer a warning if fast breathing develops. Sometimes people are unaware that they are doing it. The goal is to get the person to breathe slower — about one breath every five seconds.

When a person is hyperventilating, they should try breathing into a paper bag for five to 15 minutes so that carbon dioxide is taken back into the lungs. The bag should be held loosely over the nose and mouth. Remember that panic is one of the symptoms of hyperventilation syndrome, so reassure the person before attempting to put the paper bag over their face.

LUMP IN THROAT

The feeling of a lump in the throat is a common symptom of anxiety, particularly in young adults. The lump makes it difficult to swallow and usually comes and goes, heightened by anxiety and tension. The symptoms seem worse when the person concentrates on swallowing.

Several serious diseases can cause swallowing difficulties. In these cases, the symptoms usually develop slowly, beginning while eating solid foods, then progressively getting worse. This can result in weight loss and is more commonly seen in those over 40. Call your doctor if you develop these symptoms.

What you can do

As with any stress-related medical concern, finding the underlying cause of the anxiety is important in eliminating the symptom. Relaxation techniques may also be helpful.

Call CareWise if you would like a brochure on additional stress-reducing techniques, or would like to talk to a CareWise Nurse about stress management.

Insomnia

Having trouble getting enough sleep?

Insomnia is the inability to enjoy adequate or restful sleep. It can be defined as difficulty falling asleep, frequent awakenings during the night, or waking too early in the morning.

It's important to establish whether insomnia is *primary* (no underlying mental or physical conditions cause the problem) or *secondary* (when a physical or mental condition is responsible for the sleep disturbance).

Chronic insomnia (lasting more than a month) may be caused by depression, anxiety disorders, manic disorders, chronic pain syndromes, heart and circulation disorders, kidney disease, or *sleep apnea*, in which breathing is temporarily interrupted by airway obstruction. More than 300 over-the-counter (OTC) and prescription drugs also can contribute to insomnia including alcohol, caffeine, cardiac medications, chronic use of sleeping pills, nicotine, amphetamines and decongestants.

Behaviors that can cause or aggravate insomnia include vigorous exercise or mental exertion before bedtime, staying in bed too long in the morning or napping too much during the day.

What you can do

Practices that promote restful sleep include:

- Exercising on a regular basis (but avoiding exercise within two hours of bedtime)
- Taking a warm bath or drinking warm milk
- A regular bedtime routine that includes relaxing activities such as reading for pleasure
- Reserving the bedroom for sleeping and sex
- Avoiding alcohol and smoking before bedtime
- Drinking caffeine in moderation, before noon only
- Not napping

You can gain insights into improving your sleep by keeping a diary of your sleep patterns and behaviors.

4

know
WHAT
TO DO

Insomnia

DO THESE APPLY:

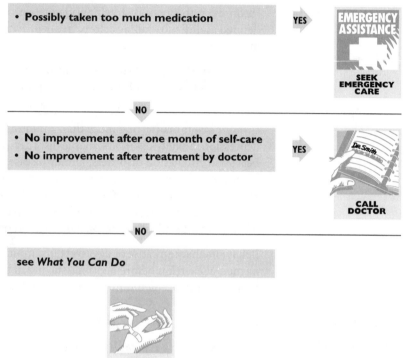

- Possibly taken too much medication

YES → **EMERGENCY ASSISTANCE**
SEEK
EMERGENCY
CARE

NO

- No improvement after one month of self-care
- No improvement after treatment by doctor

YES → *Dr. Smith*
CALL
DOCTOR

NO

see *What You Can Do*

APPLY
SELF-CARE

Depression

Treatable and worth getting help

Major depression is a potentially life-threatening physical and mental illness. The classic symptoms are a hopeless mood and a loss of pleasure in activities that used to be enjoyable. Major depression can be triggered by severe life stresses including the death of a loved one, divorce, serious financial difficulty, chronic illness and chemical dependency — particularly on alcohol or cocaine.

Limited periods of sadness and grief are a normal experience for everyone. However, the inability to recover from these episodes signals the likelihood of a potential problem for which you will want to seek some level of care.

While anyone can suffer from depression, individuals at higher risk include women, older adults and those who have a parent with a major mental illness. Women are at higher risk because pregnancy and postpartum changes can cause depression. In the elderly, poor health, social isolation, poverty and grief are factors.

While chronic illness of any sort can cause depression, some illnesses seem to have depression as one of their symptoms. These include *systemic lupus erythematosus* and *Parkinson's disease.* Certain medications, including some used to treat high blood pressure and Parkinson's disease, also can cause depression.

Unfortunately, despite gains in the past few years, a stigma is still attached to undergoing or seeking treatment for mental illness. Some people may avoid acknowledging their depression to avoid this stigma.

Children may also suffer from depression; suicide is the third leading cause of death of American teenagers.

4

Note your symptoms

Other common signs of depression include:

- Unintentional weight loss or gain

- Abnormal sleeping patterns

- Fatigue

- Feelings of worthlessness

- Excessive or inappropriate feelings of guilt

- Decreased ability to concentrate

- Recurrent thoughts of death or suicide

- A suicide attempt

- Withdrawal

- Irritability, anxiety, sadness

People with major mood swings — from depression to elation — may be suffering from a different condition known as *bipolar affective disorder*, previously called manic-depressive illness.

Another form of depression is *seasonal affective disorder*, or SAD. SAD is caused by a lack of exposure to sunlight and often occurs during the winter months in people who live in northern regions.

Symptoms can include lethargy, irritability, chronic headaches, increased appetite, weight gain and the need for more sleep. Episodes may last for several weeks.

What you can do

Major depression is a chronic, debilitating illness that can last from weeks to years. A vast majority of people who suffer from depression would benefit from some form of intervention, in the form of medication, psychotherapy (counseling) or both.

Some activities that are helpful in cases of mild depression include:

- Getting regular exercise
- Joining a support group or getting involved in group activities
- Talking to someone about your problems
- Decreasing use of alcohol or other drugs

Many SAD sufferers benefit from *phototherapy*, a medically supervised therapy which consists of daily exposure to intense full-spectrum lights (the ultraviolet wavelengths are filtered out to protect the skin). Relief usually begins in about a week. A vacation to sunnier climates, like Hawaii or the Caribbean, is a much more pleasant, but short-term solution.

Seek emergency care if you have serious thoughts of suicide, with or without a specific plan, or if you have made a suicide attempt. If someone you know has threatened suicide, take those threats seriously. Call a crisis hotline or encourage the person to seek help.

see *Know What To Do*, p. 358

know
WHAT TO DO

Depression
DO THESE APPLY:

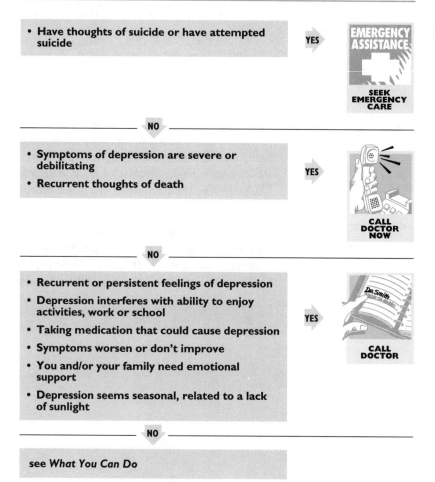

- **Have thoughts of suicide or have attempted suicide**

     YES → EMERGENCY ASSISTANCE — **SEEK EMERGENCY CARE**

— NO —

- **Symptoms of depression are severe or debilitating**
- **Recurrent thoughts of death**

     YES → **CALL DOCTOR NOW**

— NO —

- **Recurrent or persistent feelings of depression**
- **Depression interferes with ability to enjoy activities, work or school**
- **Taking medication that could cause depression**
- **Symptoms worsen or don't improve**
- **You and/or your family need emotional support**
- **Depression seems seasonal, related to a lack of sunlight**

     YES → **CALL DOCTOR**

— NO —

see *What You Can Do*

APPLY SELF-CARE

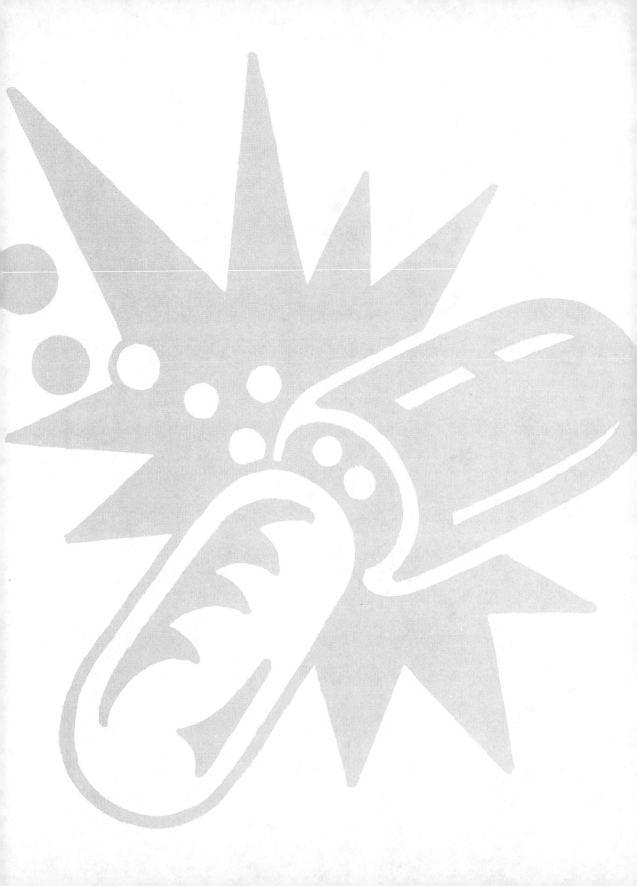

Medications

5

Using medications

Valuable tools when used wisely

When something ails us, we reach for the medicine cabinet or, if we take the complaint to a doctor, the doctor may reach for the prescription pad. Prescription and over-the-counter (OTC) drugs are a booming business, sometimes fueled by patients who feel the only way to battle an illness is with chemical bombardment.

What you can do

Prescription and nonprescription, over-the-counter (OTC) medications are valuable tools for improving and maintaining health, but they must be used cautiously and wisely. Follow these tips:

- Read the labels of prescription and over-the-counter (OTC) medications carefully to determine potential side effects and correct usage.

- Take the correct dosage of your medication.

- Pregnant or breast-feeding women, people taking an MAO inhibitor, or people being treated for serious, chronic conditions such as asthma, diabetes, epilepsy, glaucoma or heart disease should contact their doctor before taking any over-the-counter (OTC) medication.

- Never share or trade prescription drugs with anyone. The impact and side effects of drugs vary from person to person and can be unpredictable.

- Store all medications out of reach of children. If you have small children in your home, be sure all medicine bottles have safety caps.

- Take prescription medications as directed by your doctor. This may include instructions to take the medication with food, for example, or to use all the pills in a prescription even if you are feeling better after a few days.

- Make sure your doctor and pharmacist know about all the medications you are taking, to prevent a reaction between drugs.

- Throw out medications when they reach their expiration date.

- When being treated by a doctor, ask if there are treatment options that may not involve drugs, or if a less expensive but equally effective generic form of the drug is available.

A properly stocked home medicine cabinet can help you be prepared for common complaints and emergencies, and can help avoid unnecessary trips to the doctor and pharmacy. The following are some suggested items for your "home pharmacy" and first-aid kit.

Home pharmacy

Being prepared pays off

NONPRESCRIPTION DRUGS

Medication	How It Works	Risks	Comments
Antacids	Relieve heartburn or stomach upset by neutralizing acid	Some can cause constipation, others loosen stools; some brands high in sodium and should be avoided by those on low-salt diets	Avoid long-term use
Antidiarrheals	Relieve diarrhea by thickening stools and/or slowing intestinal spasms	Do not use if you have a fever; prolonged use can lead to constipation and can absorb bacteria that aid digestion	Diarrhea is body's way of flushing out infection, so use antidiarrheals only when necessary; replace body fluids depleted by diarrhea; drugs with bismuth may darken tongue or stools
Antifungal Preparations	Clear up skin fungal infections, such as athlete's foot	Few risks; preparations with selenium sulfide can burn skin if used excessively	Products with tolnaftate, clotrimazole or miconazole effective for difficult cases, but more expensive
Antihistamines/ Decongestants	Antihistamines dry mucous membranes to relieve runny nose, watery eyes and itching; decongestants shrink swollen membranes; purchase either antihistamine or decongestant, rather than a combined medication, to treat specific symptoms	Antihistamines can cause drowsiness, decongestants can cause agitation or insomnia; both can cause problems for people with certain medical conditions	Consult doctor before giving either antihistamines or decongestants to children under 12 months of age

NONPRESCRIPTION DRUGS

Medication	How It Works	Risks	Comments
Anti-inflammatories (aspirin, ibuprofen, naprosyn) (NSAIDs)	Help relieve swelling and pain in muscles and joints	Ibuprofen can pose danger to those on blood thinners; do not exceed dosage limits; aspirin can irritate stomach, cause bleeding or ulcers, and is most common cause of child poisonings; aspirin and ibuprofen should be taken with food to avoid stomach irritation **NEVER give aspirin to children/ teenagers. It can cause Reye's syndrome, a rare but often fatal condition**	Daily, low dose of aspirin may help prevent heart attack, stroke and risk of cancers in digestive system; ibuprofen available in liquid for children's use, but can upset stomach (acetaminophen is preferred medication for children); ibuprofen most effective pain reliever for menstrual cramps; naprosyn similar to ibuprofen in uses and risks
Antiseptics	Cleans wounds to prevent infection	Most are safe; hydrogen peroxide can be used to cleanse wounds	Most are of value for cleansing and are minimally effective at killing germs; soap and water can be just as useful
Cough Suppressants/ Expectorants	Suppressants control the coughing reflex to reduce dry, hacking coughs; expectorants thin mucus to make it easier to expel phlegm	Some should not be taken by people with certain health conditions; can interact with sedatives and some antidepressants; can contain alcohol	Coughs help remove phlegm to clear respiratory tract, so suppressing them may be counterproductive; products with guaifenesin are effective expectorants, those with dextromethorphan suppress coughs; call doctor before giving cough medications to children under 12 months old

NONPRESCRIPTION DRUGS

Medication	How It Works	Risks	Comments
Nasal Sprays/ Nose Drops	Shrink swollen mucous membranes to encourage free breathing; relieve runny nose and postnasal drip	Should not be used for more than three consecutive days; prolonged use can cause more swelling than before using the spray or drops	Not as effective as oral decongestants; less likely to interact with other drugs; provide temporary relief
Pain/Fever Medications (acetaminophen, aspirin, ibuprofen, naprosyn — see *Anti-inflammatories* on previous page) (NSAIDs)	Reduce fever and pain	Excessive use of acetaminophen can contribute to liver damage in heavy drinkers. **NEVER give aspirin to children/ teenagers. It can cause Reye's syndrome, a rare but often fatal condition.**	Acetaminophen is ineffective against inflammation; safest pain and fever medication for children; available in liquid form; milder to stomach than ibuprofen or aspirin; do not exceed dosage limits
Skin Irritation Medications (hydrocortisone)	Act as anti-inflammatories to temporarily relieve itching from rashes, insect bites and poison ivy	Excessive use can damage skin; generally safe if used for two weeks or less; should not be used on infected skin or near eyes	Suppress the itch reflex, but do not cure the rash; use only as much as will rub easily into skin
Laxatives	Stimulate intestines to prompt bowel movement during constipation; bulking agents soften stool to ease elimination	Few side effects if taken according to directions; regular use can decrease muscle tone and cause reliance on laxatives	Take laxatives with plenty of water; regular use can interfere with body's absorption of vitamin D and calcium

NONPRESCRIPTION DRUGS

Medication	How It Works	Risks	Comments
Syrup of Ipecac	Induces vomiting	Do not induce vomiting until a doctor or Poison Control Center directs you to do so, or if poison is petroleum-based compound (furniture polish, kerosene, gasoline) or is a strong acid or alkali (dishwasher detergent, drain opener, oven cleaner); do not use on someone who is unconscious or losing consciousness, or someone who may be susceptible to choking or inhaling into lungs; **do not give without direction to do so**	Prevent poisonings by keeping dangerous products out of your child's reach, but keep syrup of ipecac handy at all times; always call the local Poison Control Center when you suspect poisoning and follow their instructions; follow with at least 12 ounces of water and encourage the person to walk; repeat dose in 25 minutes if vomiting has not occurred; repeat only once; be alert to expiration date on container; see *Poisoning*, p. 28

First-aid supplies

Items that come in handy

In addition to over-the-counter (OTC)/nonprescription drugs, a well-stocked home medicine cabinet should include some first-aid supplies and a first-aid manual. You can put together the elements of a first-aid kit by gathering the items listed here, or you can purchase first-aid kits for your home, car, boat or other use at drugstores or through organizations such as the American Red Cross. First-aid manuals are also available at these locations.

Item	Uses
Assorted Band-Aids/Butterfly Bandages	Cover and protect small scrapes and cuts from dirt and moisture; butterfly bandages can bring edges of cut together
Tweezers	Help remove large dirt particles from wounds, slivers
Ice Bag	Reduces swelling from injuries, can provide relief from headaches
Cotton/Cotton-tipped Swabs	Useful in cleaning out wounds, lifting foreign matter from eyes; do not use inside the ear
Thermometer	Helps determine presence of fever; oral or rectal thermometers most common; electronic thermometers or ones used in child's ear are faster and easier for parents to use, but more expensive
Gauze Pads/Adhesive Tape	Fashion large bandages for wounds or scrapes that can't be covered with adhesive bandages
Sharp Scissors	Cut gauze rolls, remove jagged edges of scraped skin
Heating Pad	Speeds up healing process after swelling reduced; may relieve headaches; use on low setting
Anaphylactic Kit	To treat life-threatening allergic reactions; available by prescription from your doctor

Prevention

6

READER'S NOTE:

Prevention *is* the best medicine, which is
why we've included specific preventive
information under almost every medical
topic in *The CareWise Guide.* In addition,
this section sums up a variety of lifestyle
tips for getting and staying healthy.

6

GETTING AND STAYING HEALTHY

Health and fitness are big business in America today. But you don't have to spend a lot of money to get healthy and stay that way. Many steps toward wellness don't cost a penny.

Start by using your common sense to prevent health problems and protect yourself. For example, always use your seat belt when you're in a car and make sure you buckle your children into age-appropriate car seats. Always wear a helmet when skateboarding or riding a motorcycle, bicycle or horse.

More tips for healthy living follow. If you'd like additional information about any of them, call a CareWise Nurse and ask for a CareWise brochure on that topic.

Staying active

Crucial to good health

Exercise is a crucial element of a healthy lifestyle — no matter what your age. Regular exercise can help lower blood pressure, give you more energy, keep you fit and help you avoid serious illnesses like diabetes and coronary artery disease. It's been shown that people who exercise vigorously and regularly are more likely to cut down or stop smoking cigarettes. Exercise is also a great stress reducer.

Just 30 minutes of exercise three times a week can help you reap big health benefits, and it can be as simple as a brisk walk around the neighborhood. The key to sticking with an exercise program is choosing the type that's right for you — whether it's jogging, swimming, playing tennis, cycling or walking.

Before starting any exercise program, consult your doctor. If you've had a heart attack, surgery, joint problems or other major illness, your doctor can help you choose a program that is safe and effective.

Begin exercising gradually. Not only will this help you avoid injury, it will help you stay with your program until it eventually becomes routine. A well-rounded exercise program should include a warm-up period, moderate levels of *aerobic* exercise (heart rate is raised and sustained for a period of time to strengthen heart and lungs), strengthening exercises such as push-ups or weight training, and a cool-down period. Even during the most strenuous part of your program you should be able to talk or laugh without difficulty.

Don't be discouraged by temporary setbacks — just get back into the routine the next day. If the exercise you've chosen is too strenuous or causes injuries, slow down. Remember that if you can keep up your exercise program for a month, it will most likely become a healthful habit.

Eating right

Changes for life

Making wise food choices is an important element in a healthy lifestyle. Eating a low-fat, high-fiber, low-calorie diet also helps you maintain your proper weight. By concentrating on lifestyle changes that last a lifetime, you can avoid losing weight only to regain it a few months later.

Growing older is not an excuse for gaining extra pounds according to the new "Dietary Guidelines for Americans," released by the departments of Agriculture and Health and Human Services (1995). This means you should keep your weight within a given range for your height, rather than allowing pounds to add up with age. Weight loss should occur gradually — **one-half to one pound a week is generally safe.**

Healthy weight

Use the chart on p. 374 to evaluate your body weight. It applies to men and women of all ages, since the risks associated with excess weight appear to be the same for younger and older adults alike.

HEALTHY WEIGHT RANGES FOR MEN AND WOMEN

Height	Weight (lbs.)	Height	Weight (lbs.)	Height	Weight (lbs.)
4' 10"	91 – 119	5' 5"	114 – 150	6' 0"	140 – 184
4' 11"	94 – 124	5' 6"	118 – 155	6' 1"	144 – 189
5' 0"	97 – 128	5' 7"	121 – 160	6' 2"	148 – 195
5' 1"	101 – 132	5' 8"	125 – 164	6' 3"	152 – 200
5' 2"	104 – 137	5' 9"	129 – 169	6' 4"	156 – 205
5' 3"	107 – 141	5' 10"	132 – 174	6' 5"	160 – 211
5' 4"	111 – 146	5' 11"	136 – 179	6' 6"	164 – 216

Departments of Agriculture and Health and Human Services

Low fat

Reduce the fat in your diet by substituting fresh vegetables, graham crackers or low-fat yogurt for fat-laden snacks such as potato chips or cookies. Read food packages carefully and try to avoid buying products with more than three grams of fat per 100 calories. Eliminate fat when preparing foods by broiling, steaming or poaching instead of frying.

Good cholesterol/ bad cholesterol

Watch your cholesterol. Cholesterol has two components: low-density lipoprotein (LDL) and high-density lipoprotein (HDL). LDL is called the "bad" cholesterol because it can cause cholesterol to gather on the walls of your arteries, contributing to heart disease. HDL, the "good" cholesterol, prevents blockage of the arteries by carrying cholesterol out of the coronary artery walls. In general, your LDL should be below 130 mg/dl (milligrams per deciliter) and your HDL should be above 45 mg/dl. Your total cholesterol should be below 200 mg/dl.

Exercise and, if you smoke, start taking steps to kick the habit, to lower your LDL while raising your HDL. Also, eat foods with reduced cholesterol or less than one gram of saturated fat per 100 calories. Use fats and oils sparingly and choose those lowest in saturated fat and cholesterol: canola, corn, olive, safflower, sesame, soybean and sunflower.

Fiber and salt

Eat more fiber. The fiber in fruits, beans and peas helps lower cholesterol and reduce your risk of heart disease. Fiber in whole-grain products provides bulk to give you a "full" feeling, and helps prevent constipation.

Go easy with the salt shaker. Excess salt can raise your blood pressure and increase your risk of stroke, heart attack or kidney failure. Season foods with spices and herbs instead and watch out for high levels of salt in canned and packaged foods.

Quit smoking

It's worth it

Snuff out that cigarette. It's hard to quit smoking, but it's worth it. Within 12 hours of your last cigarette, your body begins to repair the damage to your heart and lungs. Your risk of lung cancer starts to decline about one year after you quit, and by the time you've been a nonsmoker for 10 or 15 years, your risk of cancer is about the same as for people who have never smoked.

Learn about the tools available to help you kick the habit — nicotine gum, the nicotine patch and support groups, for example. A CareWise Nurse can also help you set realistic expectations, coach you through the rough spots and offer support.

Alcohol and drugs

Monitor your use

Alcoholism, abuse of prescription or illegal drugs and chemical dependency not only harm you, they cause family problems, put unborn babies at risk for birth defects and endanger others when you drive with impaired reasoning. A CareWise Nurse can answer your questions about any kind of alcohol, drug or chemical abuse. Call for information and guidance.

6

Identify risky behaviors

Then make some changes

Does your lifestyle put your health in danger? Unprotected sex puts you at risk for HIV, the virus that causes AIDS (acquired immunodeficiency syndrome). There is no cure for this fatal disease and you can have the AIDS virus for years without having any symptoms. Using latex condoms during sex is one way to help prevent the spread of HIV. Limiting your sex partners or choosing abstinence are other options (see *HIV*, p. 344; *Safe Sex*, p. 347).

Basking in the sun or visiting the local tanning booth may give you a deep, dark tan, but these activities also put you at risk for skin cancer (see *Skin Cancer*, p. 163). Skin cancer is the most common type of cancer, but it is also the most treatable if detected early. Excessive sun exposure is usually the cause.

Skin cancers tend to develop on the face, neck and arms. Check your skin regularly for any unusual moles, spots or bumps, and contact your doctor if you notice any changes. Protect yourself by using a sunscreen with a sun protection factor (SPF) of 15 or higher; wear loose-fitting, long-sleeved clothing; and avoid going outside between 11 a.m. and 1 p.m. when the sun's rays are strongest.

> Keeping immunizations up-to-date and having appropriate diagnostic exams are also key to getting and staying healthy. Read the following pages for more important information, and call your CareWise Nurse if you have questions.

IMMUNIZATION SCHEDULE

Be smart – vaccinate

A wise health investment

Immunizations have been successful in eliminating or controlling a host of life-threatening diseases, such as smallpox, cholera and polio. This is why a thorough immunization plan — whether for your child or yourself — is an important lifetime health investment against contracting a number of serious illnesses.

To stay current on your immunizations, develop an immunization schedule with your doctor that meets your family's needs, and keep a detailed home record of vaccines.

RECOMMENDED IMMUNIZATION SCHEDULE

Age	Diphtheria Tetanus Pertussis (DTP)	Polio (OPV/IPV)	Haemophilus* Influenza b (Hib)	Hepatitis B**	Measles Mumps Rubella (MMR)	VZV*** (Chicken Pox)	Tetanus Diphtheria (Td) booster
Birth				●			
2 months	●	●	●	●			
4 months	●	●	●				
6 months	●	●	●	●			
12 months	●		●		●		
12 to 18 months						●	
4 to 6 years	●	●			● †		
11 to 12 years				● (if not immunized as an infant)	● (if not immunized as an infant)		
14 to 16 years							● ‡
Over 65 years	Pneumococcal vaccine (one time only in most cases); flu vaccine (annually)						

*Given at 6 and/or 12 months, depending on brand of Hib vaccine.

**There are several possible schedules for hepatitis B immunization.

***Teens and adults who have never had chicken pox should receive two doses given four to eight weeks apart.

†Where required by public health authorities for school entry; otherwise given at 11-12 years old. Check with your doctor.

‡ If you get a dirty wound and have not had a tetanus booster within the last five years, your doctor will probably recommend an injection. Vaccinate every 10 years throughout adulthood.

SCREENING GUIDELINES

Catching problems early

An ounce of prevention . . .

It's a fact that some medical tests are unnecessary, costly and over-prescribed. Yet others can play an important role in increasing your longevity and quality of life, while saving thousands — or even hundreds of thousands — of dollars in the long run by catching a potentially serious problem early.

Here are a few of the preventive tests that are recommended for healthy adults. If you have a serious medical condition or other high-risk factors, consult your doctor about other necessary tests, or more frequent tests. **Infants, children and pregnant women also need other types of tests.**

Exam	Who Needs It	How Often
Blood Pressure Measurement	All adults	Every two years for healthy adults
Cholesterol Screening (to detect high blood cholesterol levels, which may lead to atherosclerosis)	All adults, most important for middle-aged men, anyone with history of heart disease, or smokers	Every five years
Pap Smear (to detect cervical cancer)	All women beginning at age 18 or at onset of sexual activity	Annually if there is a history of STDs or multiple sex partners, or every three years after two normal annual exams
Mammogram	All women beginning at age 50, or at age 35 if a family history of premenopausal breast cancer in mother or sister	Every one to two years on doctor's advice

Exam	Who Needs It	How Often
Professional Breast Exam	All women during routine checkup and annually after age 40; beginning annually at age 35 if a family history of premenopausal breast cancer in mother or sister	During routine checkup every one to two years at age 18; annually after age 40; (a monthly self-exam is also recommended)*
Sigmoidoscopy (to detect colon/rectal cancer)	Everyone over age 50 with inflammatory bowel disease, colon polyps or family history of colon cancer	Every five years or on doctor's advice
Fecal Occult Blood Testing (stool test for early detection of colon/rectal cancer)	Same as for sigmoidoscopy	The American Cancer Society, American College of Gastroenterology and the National Cancer Institute recommend annual testing for people with no symptoms or on doctor's advice
Digital Rectal Exam (to detect prostate cancer) Test is not sensitive enough to detect prostate cancer reliably; prostate enlargement can be detected by this test	The American Cancer Society and the National Cancer Institute recommend an annual exam after age 40 for all men	Insufficient evidence for all experts to recommend for or against routine testing of men with no symptoms
Glaucoma Screen	Everyone over age 40	Every two years or on doctor's advice
Electrocardiogram or EKG (to detect coronary artery disease)	Not recommended for routine screening of people without symptoms	
Exercise Stress Test (to screen for heart disease)	Men over 40 who have two or more major risk factors for heart disease (high cholesterol, high blood pressure, smoking, diabetes, family history of early onset of heart disease)	Selectively on doctor's advice
Chest X-ray	Not recommended as routine screening of people without symptoms	Selectively on doctor's advice
Common Lab Tests (CBC, urinalysis, glucose, thyroid, liver, kidney, syphilis, tuberculin)	Not recommended as routine screening of people without symptoms	Selectively on doctor's advice

*see *Breast Self-Exam*, p. 308

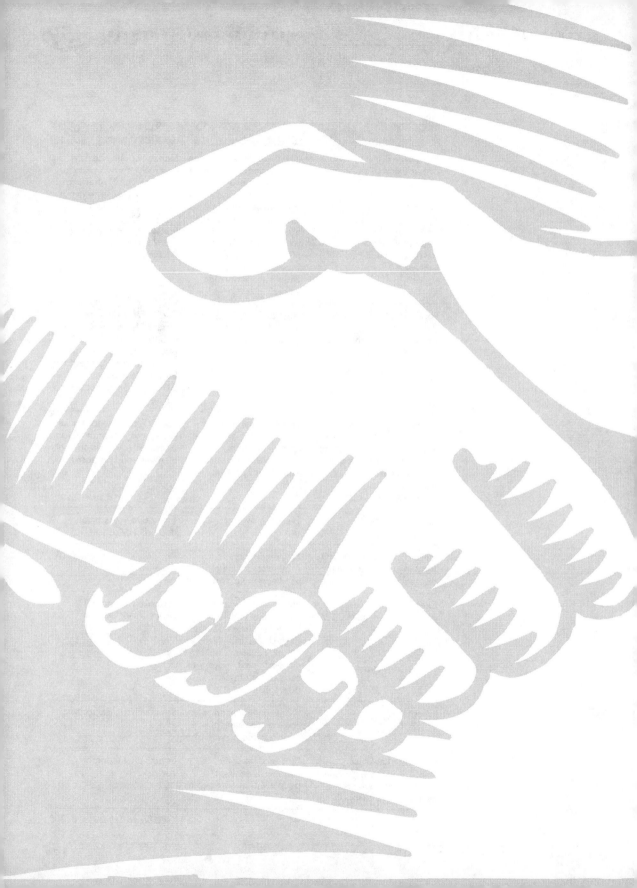

Working with your doctor

Finding the right doctor

A few tips on the selection process

The first step toward getting the best and most appropriate health care is finding a doctor you feel comfortable with and can work with on a long-term basis. Here are a few tips for evaluating and choosing a doctor.

Decide what type of doctor you need

It is usually best to select a primary care doctor who can take care of most of your routine medical concerns and refer you to a specialist, if necessary. Look for someone who is certified in family practice (FP), general practice (GP), internal medicine (IM), or pediatrics (for children).

Because some family practitioners, general practitioners and internists do not provide routine gynecologic or obstetric care, it may be necessary to select a gynecologist/obstetrician for women's health concerns.

Find a few doctors to choose from

Ask your friends and family, or other health professionals you may know, for their recommendations. Or call your employer's health plan office for suggestions. Some health care plans, such as health maintenance organizations (HMOs), may provide assistance in selecting a doctor. If your insurance plan covers a limited list of doctors, ask them to send you the list to help you make a decision.

Call the doctor's office and ask questions

After you have identified a few potential doctors, call their offices and ask some questions. Tell the receptionist you want to find a doctor for your ongoing care and are wondering if the doctor is accepting new patients. If the answer is yes, ask if you can get some additional information. Also, if you have children, ask about age limitations (some GPs and internists take only adult patients).

Questions you might want to ask include:

- Is the doctor board certified in your state? If so, in what specialty?

- Does he or she have practice privileges at accredited hospitals? (If the answer is yes, this indicates that the doctor's credentials have been screened by the hospitals and tells you which facilities would be used if you were hospitalized.)

- If you belong to a managed care organization, is the doctor a member of that organization? Your insurance may not cover services provided by nonmember doctors.

- Where is the doctor's office located and what are the office hours?

- If you call about an urgent medical problem, will you be seen the same day? What is the average waiting time for a nonurgent appointment?

- What kind of back-up is provided when the doctor is unavailable?

- Is the doctor willing to discuss medical problems over the phone with you? If so, is there a charge?

- Are other medical services (x-rays, laboratory tests, etc.) readily available when needed?

- Is the doctor eligible for maximum payments under your health plan?

- What is the cost of an average office visit?

- Does the doctor's office require payment at each visit?

- What are the terms of payment? Is there a finance charge?

Next, schedule an office visit

Once you find a doctor who seems like a good candidate, schedule an appointment. (Call a CareWise Nurse before the appointment if you'd like help preparing a list of questions for the doctor, tailored to your specific medical concerns.)

During the appointment, note whether the doctor:

- Listens to your concerns and obtains a thorough history of your problem

- Answers your questions and explains the treatment plan completely, in terms you can understand

- Discusses treatment alternatives with you and goes over the risks and benefits

- Is willing to make a referral to a specialist if he or she cannot readily diagnose or treat your condition

- Seems aware of cost as well as quality of care

- Is responsive when you express your fears, concerns and preferences

- Is someone you feel you can talk to and work with in the months and years to come

After the visit, check your bills

- Are the bills or insurance claims processed promptly and accurately?

- Are the charges detailed and readily identifiable? Are there any unexpected or unexplained charges?

- If the doctor's office handles your insurance claims, are they submitted to the insurance company in a timely manner?

- If you must handle the insurance claims yourself, is the doctor's office willing to assist you and provide whatever additional documentation may be required?

Becoming partners with your doctor

It definitely pays off

Many of us tend to believe that we have little or nothing to contribute to our own treatment program. But think again. Each of us is the one-and-only possible expert when it comes to:

- Our family history
- Our symptoms and how they developed
- Our opinions about what has and hasn't worked for us in the past
- How we feel about various treatment options
- Our lifestyle and the things that are important to us
- Our preferences, concerns and fears

Doctors report that 70% of their correct diagnoses are the result of information provided by the patient. What's more, statistics show that patients who speak up, share information, ask questions and participate in treatment decisions enjoy a noticeable improvement in the quality and appropriateness of their care.

So how do you go about becoming an effective partner with your doctor?

Between doctor visits

- Learn to observe your own body and keep a record of your symptoms and concerns so that you're ready to report accurate information to your doctor. For example:

  - **Be able to give your doctor an exact temperature reading** — and ready to report whether it's an oral, *axillary* (taken in the armpit) or rectal temperature. This is much more helpful than saying that you or a member of your family is "burning up." If you don't have a thermometer, buy one and learn to use it.

  - **Learn to measure pulse rate and its regularity**. Whether you are worried about a feverish child or a spouse who is experiencing heart palpitations, measuring the person's pulse — which means counting the number of heartbeats in one minute — and noticing whether the rhythm of the beats is regular or irregular, can provide your doctor with useful information (see *Pulse* in Index).

- **For women over age 18, make a habit of examining your breasts once a month**. Learn what is normal and customary for you and report any changes — such as unusual lumps or thickening — to your doctor (see *Breast Lumps*, p. 306). Once males are in their teens, they should begin examining their penis and testes each month for any changes that could indicate infection or cancer (see *Genital Health*, p. 328).

- **Know what your normal weight is**. If it changes, keep track of how much and over what period of time. Knowing about any sudden weight loss or gain can help your doctor diagnose certain illnesses. (Call CareWise for more information or material on weight, exercise and healthy diets.)

- **Become familiar with your skin** — moles, warts, bruises, birthmarks, etc., as well as overall tone and color. Learn to notice and track anything unusual — a mole that is growing or a sore that isn't healing — that may need immediate attention.

In short, get to know your whole body — from head to toe — so you will know what is normal for you. Keep a list of any changes, symptoms or areas of concern and bring it with you to your next doctor visit.

• For nonemergencies, check this book or call CareWise before calling your doctor. You may discover some self-care options that can save the time and expense of a doctor visit.

• If you decide to go to the doctor, prepare for the visit. Give some careful thought to your most important health concerns. Get ready to describe them — in order of importance — as completely and concisely as possible. Write down names of your medications and questions you want to ask your doctor (if you would like help developing questions, call CareWise).

At the doctor's office . . .

Begin the conversation with the topics you are *most* worried about — not your minor complaints — and be as honest and direct as possible about your feelings and concerns. Keep it short and to the point, but take the time you need to describe your problem.

Taking an active role

Whether your doctor suggests putting you on medication, running a few tests, or scheduling a minor procedure or major surgery — it *always* pays off to find out what's going on and participate in the decision-making process.

Yes, your doctor has years of training and offers invaluable medical advice. But only you can really decide if the benefits outweigh the risks — for your particular situation — and if the treatment plan is something you can live with and incorporate into your lifestyle.

TAKING AN ACTIVE ROLE IN TREATMENT DECISIONS

- Ask your doctor to explain the various treatment options — along with the benefits, risks and costs of each — before going ahead with *anything*: "What is the official name of the test/procedure/ medication?" "Why do I need it?" "What will the procedure involve?" "What are the risks and benefits?" "How much will it cost?" "What are the alternatives?" "Would it be possible to just watch and wait for a while?" Take notes if it helps.

- If you don't understand your doctor's explanations, be persistent and ask again: "Could you go over that part again?" "Do you have any material I can read at home?" "Can you show me on paper what will happen?"

- If a prescription drug is suggested, ask about the side effects, and the possibility of using a less expensive but effective generic substitute.

- If a major test or surgery is recommended, ask if there are other treatment options that are equally effective, or if you can watch and wait for a while without putting your health at risk.

- Ask if there will be any restrictions on activity and, if so, how long the restrictions will be necessary. If some treatment is suggested that you know you just can't or won't be able to handle — "I have three kids at home! I can't stay in bed all day!" — speak up. Chances are you and your doctor can work out a suitable alternative.

- Find out if there is anything else — besides or in addition to a prescription or treatment — you can do for *yourself* to help the problem or speed your recovery.

7

Sorting through your options

- If it's a nonemergency, don't rush into anything! Remember that very few medical procedures are actually emergencies. There is usually time to think about the options and select the one that seems best for you.

- Call CareWise if you'd like help understanding your medical problem, evaluating options for care, planning questions for your doctor — or if you just want someone to talk to about your health concern. As needed, CareWise Nurses can send you current medical material available in print — tailored to meet your specific needs and level of understanding.

- If you find you have more questions for your doctor, or need additional information, call your doctor's office and ask!

Once treatment is decided . . .

- Make sure you understand all the treatment instructions. If not, ask more questions!

- **Carefully follow your treatment program**. For example, write down your medication schedule and each time you take the medicines. Always fully comply with all instructions, and always talk to your doctor before altering your treatment or medication program.

- Keep track of any side effects and call your doctor or CareWise if you are worried or have any questions, or if something doesn't seem right (see *Using Medications*, p. 362).

CONSIDERING SURGERY? CALL CAREWISE!

Deciding whether or not to have nonemergency surgery can be tough, and it pays to get as much information as you can before making the decision. A CareWise Nurse will be glad to help you prepare a list of questions for your surgeon that's tailored to meet your specific concerns and questions. Just call!

Index

B

Baby
    See specific topic; **Childhood
    diseases/concerns**
Baby rashes, *chart* **82**
    See also **Rashes**
Back pain
    described **274 - 277**
    spine, *illustrated* 274, 276
    See also **Muscle/bone/joint
    concerns; Neck injury;
    Spinal injury**
Bacterial infections. *See specific
    medical topic*
Barotitis 195, 196
Bedbugs 156 - 157
Bee stings 53, **55 - 56, 58 - 59**
Benadryl 140
Benign, *defined* 306
Benign fibrocystic breasts
    defined 306
Benign prostatic hypertrophy
    described **331 - 334**
Biopsy, *defined* **164**
Bipolar affective disorder
    defined 356
    See also **Depression; Mental
    health**
Birth control
    methods, *chart* **336 - 338**
Birth-control pills, *chart* **337**
Bismuth 364
Bites
    allergic reaction 53, 56,
    58 - 59
    animal bites **53 - 54**, 58 - 59
    human bites **53 - 54**, 58 - 59
    hydrocortisone cream **366**
    infection from **53 - 54,
    58 - 59**

insect bites **55 - 56, 58 - 59**
snakebites **57 - 59**
spider bites **55, 58 - 59**
tetanus booster 53, **377**
tick bites **158 - 160**
Blackheads 127, 137
Blackout. *See* **Unconsciousness**
Bladder. *See* **Urinary problems
(men) (women)**
Bleeding
    controlling severe **47**, 77
    pressure points **47**
    gastrointestinal bleeding
    symptom of 252
    head/spinal injury
    symptom of **60, 63**
    See also **Menstrual cycle;
    Painful periods; Uterine
    bleeding**
Blisters
    burns, symptom of **30**
    chicken pox
    symptom of **83**
    frostbite, symptom of
    37, 39
    genital herpes **341 - 343**
    impetigo, symptom of 127,
    144 - 145
    oral herpes **200**, 341
Blood clots
    leg pain and **283 - 284, 286**
Blood pressure
    examination schedule
    chart **378**
    See also **Hypertension**
Bloody stools 256, 261
Bloody urine
    kidney stones, symptom
    of 267
    prostate cancer, symptom
    of 333 - 334

rapid
  shock, symptom of **43**
slowing
  hypothermia, symptom of
  37, 39
  shock, symptom of **43**
weak
  shock, symptom of **43**
Punctures
  described **50 - 52**
  tetanus booster 50, **377**
  See also **Abrasions; Cuts;**
    Fishhooks; Splinters;
    Wounds
Pupil change
  head/spinal injury
    symptom of **61**, 63
  shock, symptom of **43**
  stress, symptom of 349
Pus. *See* **Infected wounds; Skin**
  concerns; Vaginal discharge

Q

Quick reference **v**

R

Rabies 53 - 54
Rashes
  baby, *chart* **82**
  childhood rashes, *chart* **82**
  human immunodeficiency
    virus (HIV),
    symptom of **344**
  hydrocortisone cream
    chart **366**

skin symptoms
  chart **127 - 129**
  See also specific topic
Rectal/anal concerns
  anal warts 151
  digital rectal exam
    chart **379**
  fecal occult blood testing
    chart **379**
  hemorrhoids 257
  hydrocortisone cream
    257, **366**
  rectum, *illustrated* 329
  sigmoidoscopy, *chart* **379**
  See also **Abdominal/**
    gastrointestinal
    concerns
Red measles. *See* **Measles**
Referred pain, *defined* 274
Reflux, *defined* 251
Renal concerns. *See specific*
  topic; Kidneys; **Urinary**
  problems (men) (women)
Respiratory concerns
  antihistamines/
    decongestants, *chart* **364**
  asthma **213 - 215**
  bronchitis **228 - 229**
  chest pain **218 - 221**
  chest x-ray **379**
  colds 174, **182 - 184**
  cough suppressants/
    expectorants, *chart* **365**
  croup **100 - 102**
  emphysema **232 - 234**
  hyperventilation syndrome
    219, 351
  influenza **230 - 231**
  pneumococcal vaccine
    chart **377**
  pneumonia **235 - 237**

Y

Yeast infections
    described   322 - 324
    vaginal discharge   **322 - 324**
    See also Vaginal concerns

Z

Zeasorb-AF   148